Dental Surgery Assistants' Handbook

Second Edition

† University of Bristol Dental School and Hospital
  Lower Maudlin Street, Bristol, BS1 2LY, United Kingdom

* Examiner for the National Certificate of the Examining Board for Dental Surgery Assistants, United Kingdom

DENTAL SURGERY ASSISTANTS' HANDBOOK

SECOND EDITION

Roger G Smith* BChD, MDS, FDSRCS Eng.
Consultant Senior Lecturer in Periodontology†

Diane Bell * RDSA, FETC, DipDHE
Senior Tutor Dental Surgery Assistant†

Graham R Hooper BDS
General Dental Practitioner

Robin W Matthews BDS, PhD, MDS
Senior Lecturer in Oral Medicine, Pathology and Microbiology†

Stephen R Porter BSc, MBChB, FDSRCS, FDSRCSE, PhD
Lecturer in Oral Medicine, Pathology and Microbiology†

Crispian Scully PhD, MD, MDS, FDSRCPS, FFDRCSI, FDSRCS, FRCPath
Professor of Oral Medicine, Pathology and Microbiology†

D Keith Stables* BDS, DDPHRCS Eng.
Senior Dental Officer, Avon Community Dental Services
Clinical Teacher in Child Dental Health (Paediatric Dentistry)†

Christopher D Stephens BDS, MDS, FDSRCSE, MOrthRCS Eng.
Professor of Child Dental Health†

Adrian C Watkinson BChD, MDS, FDSRCSE, DRDRCSE
Lecturer in Prosthodontics†

M Mosby

St. Louis Baltimore Boston Chicago London Philadelphia Sydney Toronto

ISBN 1-56375-622-6

Cataloguing in Publication Data
CIP catalogue records for this book are available from the British
Library and the US Library of Congress.

Publisher:	Fiona Foley
Project managers:	Claire Hooper
	Moira Sarsfield
Design:	Pete Wilder
Illustration:	Marion Tasker
Production:	Susan Bishop

Originated by Mandarin Offset (HK) Ltd.
Produced by China Translation and Printing Services Ltd.
Printed and bound in Hong Kong, 1993
Typeset in Galliard and Helvetica

Preface

There was a very encouraging response to the First Edition of the *Dental Surgery Assistants' Handbook*, published in 1988.

Since that time various changes have occurred in the practice of Dentistry which affect DSAs, not least the growing recognition of the crucial role any DSA has in ensuring the success of any dental practice. Success can of course be measured in various ways. In this Edition, as in the First Edition, we are primarily focusing on the well-being of the many patients whom we see, who together may have various oral and dental, and sometimes medical, problems requiring a whole range of appropriate care. The DSA thus requires a broad understanding of dental and oral diseases and their management.

We hope that each section benefits by being written, as previously, by people with a depth of knowledge and interest in their area. Also, each section is designed to be self-contained, and for this reason we have followed our reviewers' helpful suggestion by putting *"Instructions to patients"* and *"Instrument lay-ups"* in the sections to which they belong instead of collecting them together at the end. However, we have increased cross-references between chapters, and we are grateful to our Publishers for allowing us a much-expanded Index; we hope that both measures will assist readers who wish to pursue topics which appear in several sections.

Most chapters have been expanded to take account of recent changes. Mrs Diane Bell has revised and amalgamated chapters 1 and 16 which were contributed to the first Edition by Mrs Kathleen Holden. Chapter 9 has been substantially rewritten, sections on Conscious Sedation and Implants have been added to Chapters 12 and 14 respectively, and various other important additions, alterations and corrections have been made in all the remaining chapters.

We need to emphasise again that practical skills cannot be acquired merely from books and that these can only be developed at the chairside under the guidance of Dental Surgeons, who may have their own preferences for managing clinical procedures in particular ways.

Post-qualification training is further enhancing the work and status of DSAs. Other changes may be expected to flow in the UK from the Nuffield Enquiry into the Training and Education of Personnel Auxiliary to Dentistry (which is awaited as we go to print) and the NVQ system of qualification.

In the First Edition we used the abbreviation ' DSA' meaning ' Dental Surgery Assistant' but implying such equivalent personnel as Dental Nurses and Chairside Assistants. After much consideration we have decided to retain the term 'DSA' in the Second Edition (it has the merit of being easily seen on the page!) although we realise that the term Dental Nurse may soon gain wider usage (and may even influence the title of a Third Edition!)

I wish to express my gratitude to my colleagues again for their willing collaboration, to Mrs Gillian Key (Tutor DSA: Bristol Dental Hospital) and Mrs Jennifer Lavery (The Secretary: National Examining Board for Dental Surgery Assistants) for their kind advice and help, and to our DSAs and secretaries who have assisted us. And our particular thanks to the staff at Gower Medical Publishing for their superb presentation.

Roger G Smith
Bristol , April 1993

Contents

1. The DSA in the Dental Environment

QUALITIES OF A DSA
Personality
You should have a friendly and approachable manner whilst at all times maintaining a professional attitude. A sense of humour and ability to put people at ease would both be assets.

Personal problems and views (e.g. political) should not be discussed at the surgery. Social small talk with colleagues should be kept out of patients' hearing. You should avoid arguments with patients. Also, patients sometimes give information which must be treated with strict confidence; to break this confidentiality would be an offence and could lead to instant dismissal. Matters concerning patients or patient management should never be discussed with other patients or outside the practice. Patients who ask to see their dental records should be referred to the Dentist.

Appearance
In your uniform, you are seen by the public as a nurse. Some guidelines on appearance are as follows:

- Hair should preferably be short or off the collar; long hair should be tied back neatly.

- Nails should be short and clean. Any nail varnish should not be coloured.

- Make-up, if used, should be minimal with subtle colours.

- Perfumes or similar substances should be light.

- Jewellery should be limited to a wrist watch and one plain ring.

- Earrings if worn should be of a small stud type; 'drop earrings' can be dangerous (they may touch the patients or may be grabbed by patients during uncontrolled movements).

- The uniform (tunic top and trousers or skirt, or dress) should be clean and smart; dresses or skirts should be knee-length.

- Shoes should have closed-in toes for comfort and protection (from falling instruments).

Clearly several of the above recommendations are made from considerations of health and safety.

Communication skills
The DSA must be able to communicate effectively with other members of the dental team (the Dental Surgeon, Dental Hygienist, Receptionist, Practice Manager, and Dental Technician).

As good communication with all patients and callers to the dental surgery is of the utmost importance, a variety of good communication skills are essential to ensure smooth running of the practice.

Speech
You should aim to speak clearly and without jargon. Some patients may be hard of hearing or their first language may not be yours; some patients may need details repeating. Patience and tact with patients are good qualities to be cultivated.

You will learn many professional words, which you should generally avoid using with patients who may not understand them (or may even misunderstand them).

Telephone
The telephone message which you receive may be the first contact which the caller has with your surgery. As first impressions count, you should answer with a clear voice, stating the name of the surgery or dentist(s). Calls should be answered promptly and the caller dealt with in a pleasant but efficient and courteous manner. Messages should be written down, particularly if they are to be passed to someone else at the surgery.

Written messages
As you may be required to contact patients by letter (e.g. to alter appointments or to send accounts), your handwriting should be neat and legible. There should be no spelling mistakes in the message, the address (and postcode), or patient's name.

Computer skills
As a number of dental surgeries have installed a computer system for patients' appointments and stock control, a knowledge of computers may be useful but is not essential.

TRAINING AND CAREER PROSPECTS
Training
Although it is not essential for a DSA to gain a qualification, you would be strongly advised to consider the benefits of doing so. The course of training

leading to a qualification will give you a better understanding of dentistry, which in turn will make your work far more rewarding, as you will be able to contribute more effectively and confidently in the care and management of patients.

A variety of training programmes are available as outlined below. It would be advisable to contact your choice of training scheme early to check on any entrance requirements or restrictions (some courses have age restrictions or educational requirements).

Some centres which offer training courses conduct their own end-of-course qualifying examination which leads to the award of a certificate and badge.

However, the majority of dental nurses in the UK and Eire will (also) wish to obtain the *National Certificate for Dental Surgery Assistants*. It would be advisable at an early stage to obtain the relevant syllabus and regulations (from the Examining Board for Dental Surgery Assistants; the address is on page 20) which should be studied in conjunction with the report of the Dental Surgery Assistants Standards and Training Advisory Board (DSASTAB) from the Association of Dental Surgery Assistants (address on page 20).

The NVQ system of qualification is under active consideration.

Training programmes are as follows:

- Full-time courses, mostly provided by Dental Schools and Hospitals listed on page XX, but some are in Colleges of Further Education and in the Armed Forces.

- Evening Classes, mostly held in Colleges of Further Education. In order to be eligible for such courses, you need to be employed by a Dental Surgeon. The National Examining Board, or Careers Office of your Local Authority, will be able to tell you if such a course is available in your area.

- Day Release courses, which are usually restricted to Youth Training Schemes available to young people between 16 and 18 years of age. Local Authority Careers Offices should have full details.

Areas of employment
General dental practice
Some surgeries are NHS, others are private, and some are both. Some practices are restricted to Orthodontics, Oral Surgery, or other specialist treatment. Vacancies for dental nurses may be advertised in local papers.

Community dental health service
Such surgeries provide NHS dentistry which is limited to children, expectant mothers, handicapped people, and the elderly. Local papers may advertise suitable vacancies.

Hospital service
Teaching hospitals provide NHS dentistry and specialist care. Some general hospitals incorporate Units specialising in Oral and Facio-Maxillary Surgery, Orthodontics, and Restorative Dentistry (Conservation, Periodontology, Prosthetics). Newspapers may advertise suitable vacancies, or enquiries may be made to the Administrative Offices of specific hospitals.

Career prospects
Qualification may open the way, usually after a minimum of 3 post-qualification years of work, to more senior positions in dental nursing in any of the above situations. Some DSAs go on to be *Practice Managers* or *Tutors,* although both require further training, the latter requiring a *City and Guilds Further Adult Education Teaching Certificate.*

To become a *Dental Health Educator* requires a further one year's training at a College of Further Education, usually at evening classes, or on a day-release course.

To become a *Dental Hygienist* requires further training of up to 2 years in a Dental Teaching Hospital or in the Armed Forces. This training is restricted to qualified dental nurses who also have a minimum of five passes at GCSE level (including English and Human Biology).

Post-qualification courses
Courses for qualified DSAs, whose name appears in the voluntary Dental Surgery Assistants' Register (page 20), are available in:

- Conscious Sedation and Resuscitation

- Oral Health Education

- Dental Radiography

Certificates are issued upon satisfactory completion of any of these courses. The Association of Dental Surgery Assistants (page XX) will have information on any courses in your area.

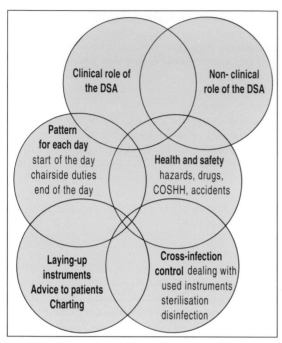

Fig. 1.1 *The overlapping areas of responsibility of the DSA.*

ROLE OF THE DSA

As Fig 1.1 shows, the dental nurse has many overlapping responsibilities. The various clinical duties regarding the running of the surgery and the proper care of patients have to be carried out with due regard to cross-infection control and health and safety requirements. Equally, health and safety considerations govern certain non-clinical duties. Throughout the sections which follow, their interdependence needs to be borne in mind.

• Clinical Role of the DSA

Pattern for each day
Start of the day
At the beginning of each day the DSA should put on a clean uniform and go through the following procedure to prepare the dental surgery for patients:

1. Switch on ventilators, heaters, air conditioners as necessary.

2. Switch on all appliances (steriliser, compressor, dental chair, suction apparatus) and check that they are in good working order.

3. Check the stock of dental materials and drugs

(e.g. local anaesthetic cartridges, medications).

4. Ensure that emergency drugs and equipment (page 158) are readily available and in working order.

5. Provide a clean coat for the dentist, and check soap, towels, skin cleanser, protective gloves and eye wear for use by staff in the surgery.

6. Waiting areas and toilets used by patients should be checked for cleanliness and tidiness and that all necessary facilities are provided.

7. Consult the day list for any special requirements (e.g. patients in wheelchairs, laboratory work).

8. Ensure that the notes, charts, and correct radiographs of all patients expected are to hand.

9. Ensure that all appropriate instruments are sterile and ready for use.

10. Provide a mouthwash, bib, tissues, and protective eye wear for the first patient.

Chairside duties
You should greet all patients with a smile and a friendly manner, assisting them to the dental chair and adjusting it for their comfort and in accordance with the dentist's requirements. It is clearly essential to check the patient's identity and that the records to hand are those of the patient. Each patient should be provided with a protective bib, clean mouthwash, protective eyewear, tissues, and a small bowl containing mouthwash for any dentures or appliances being worn.

It is important to remain in the surgery whilst the dentist is treating patients to give them reassurance, comfort and care, as well as assisting the dentist in the procedure being performed. The DSA is also a witness to what is said and done in the surgery. Patients welcome the DSA's help in removing any blood or debris from around the mouth at the end of the procedure.

To fulfil these obligations, the dentist will expect of the DSA the following:

- to be attentive and alert at all times

- to become familiar with the different instruments and their uses (appropriate lists of instruments are given in the relevant sections of the book see page 13).

- to learn the various procedures and to anticipate what instruments will be needed in sequence, handing the right instrument to the dentist at the correct time and perhaps receiving another.

- to place suction tips correctly and effectively as required.

- to learn dental terminology, and be able to chart teeth correctly (examples of charts are shown later in this chapter and in Chapter 9).

- to instruct patients (page 13).

- to mix materials according to manufacturers' recommendations.

- to assist with X-ray films (page 17).

- to be trained to assist in emergency procedures.

In between each patient the DSA should carefully remove all instruments, handpieces, burs and 3-in-1 tips from the chairside to the cleaning and sterilising area (page 12). The spittoon should be cleaned and work surfaces, light switches, and controls should be wiped with a suitable disinfectant. The DSA should also ensure that the dentist writes up the patient's treatment in the file. Before the next patient enters the surgery, the DSA should put out:

- sterile instruments and 3-in-1 tips as required.

- mouthwash and bib.

- protective eyewear for patient, dentist, and nurse.

- gloves and masks for dentist and nurse.

- the correct records for the patient.

End of the day
The following duties should be performed before closing the surgery:

1. The surgery should be cleaned as one would between patients.

2. Clean the suction tubes and filters following manufacturers' specifications.

3. Turn off all appliances.

4. Check that all records have been correctly written up by the dentist, before all notes, forms and X-ray films are transferred to the Receptionist for processing.

5. Put away correctly all sterile instruments and handpieces.

6. Ensure that all impressions etc., have been put ready for transferring to the laboratory.

7. Check the patients' list for the next working day for any special needs or arrangements.

8. Leave the surgery clean and tidy.

Cross-infection control
It is important that the DSA understands the meaning of the terms sterilisation and disinfection:

Sterilisation is the process of killing all living microorganisms, bacteria, spores, viruses, and fungi.

Disinfection is the process of killing bacteria and fungi, but not spores and viruses (hepatitis B is a virus).

Sterilisation of instruments is carried out to prevent *cross-infection* which is the transfer of microorganisms from one person to another, for example, from Dental Surgeon to patient, patient to Dental Surgeon, and DSA to Dental Surgeon and patient.

Guidelines to reduce the risk of cross infection in the dental surgery are as follows:

- The Dental Surgeon and DSA must be inoculated against hepatitis B virus.

- The patient's medical history (page 54) should be regularly updated by the dentist.

- Treat all saliva and blood as infected; treat every patient with extreme care and maintain high standards of cleanliness and sterilisation procedures to ensure safety for everyone.

- Always wear gloves when treating patients and preferably change them after each patient (or wash and dry them thoroughly between each patient).

- Always wear a face mask and protective eye wear

when using instruments which may cause a spray (3-in-1 syringe, ultrasonic scaler or air rotor hand piece).

- Ensure that all instruments are sterile for every patient (replace ones provided for a patient but not used).

- All handpieces, 3-in-1 tips and burs should be changed between patients, providing sterile replacements for the next patient.

- Use disposable items where possible, e.g. bibs, mouthwash cups.

- Instruments, handpieces, burs and 3-in-1 tips should be removed after use for cleaning and sterilising.

Dealing with used instruments

As stated earlier, after each patient has been treated the DSA should carefully remove from the chairside to the cleaning and sterilising area all used instruments, handpieces, burs, and 3-in-1 tips. As this equipment may be contaminated with saliva and blood, the following procedure is then advised.

Whilst wearing heavy duty rubber gloves, carefully remove all 'sharps' (needles and blades) and place them in a 'sharps' container, and place other disposable items in appropriate containers. Thoroughly scrub all instruments in running warm water or place them in an ultrasonic water bath; rinse thoroughly after cleaning and place into a steriliser and activate the cycle (see next section).

Wipe handpieces with disinfectant before spraying them with oil and sterilising them according to the manufacturers' specifications. Clean burs with a bur brush before sterilising them in a suitable chemical.

Place disposable items stained with potentially infected substances (e.g. blood, pus) in a specially designated waste disposal bag, and similarly stained non-disposable items (e.g. operating gowns) in another special bag for the laundry.

Place waste amalgam in an unbreakable pot with a watertight lid, containing sufficient 2% potassium permanganate or water to cover the material (see page 62).

Methods of sterilisation
Autoclave
This is the most reliable method of sterilisation. Steam under pressure kills all bacteria, spores, viruses and fungi, if the correct temperature and pressure is reached and maintained for 3 minutes.

Directions for using an autoclave
- The instruments, after washing and rinsing, should be placed on to the trays which fit inside the autoclave.

- Ensure that there is sufficient distilled water in the water tank.

- Close the door *tightly* and activate the cycle.

- The water is then heated to a temperature of 134°C and the pressure reaches 32lb per sq inch, which is maintained for 3 minutes (and is known as the 'sterilisation time').

- After sterilisation, condensing occurs, when the temperature and pressure drop.

- The whole cycle takes about 15–20 minutes; after the cycle is completed, a light will indicate that the door can be opened.

- The instruments inside will be hot, so great care must be taken when removing them.

Hot air oven
Instruments placed in this steriliser must be washed as before, but then dried before placing in the oven (to prevent rusting).

- The instruments are placed on a tray.

- The oven, which is powered by electricity, must be switched on, and a temperature of 160°C must be reached.

- The instruments are then placed inside.

- Once the door is opened the temperature drops, so it is very important that a temperature of 160°C is reached again before the timing starts.

This is a very slow method of sterilisation (at 160°C the sterilisation time is one hour; when the time for heating up is taken into consideration, a cycle can take up to one hour and 30 minutes to complete).

Chemical sterilisation

The most frequently used chemicals are hypochlorite and glutaraldehyde. Plastic items and other instruments unable to withstand heat can be sterilised by these chemicals, if left totally immersed for 8 hours; any less than this will only disinfect them. When instruments are removed the chemical must be thoroughly rinsed off using distilled water. Chemicals of this type can be hazardous if not handled correctly (page 19).

Industrial sterilisation

This method, which uses gamma radiation (active agent Cobalt 60), is used in industry to sterilise bulk disposable items, e.g. scalpel blades, needles, sutures, etc., and is not found in dental surgeries or hospitals.

Methods for disinfecting instruments
Hand pieces

Many makes are now able to withstand the high temperatures of an autoclave. A sterile handpiece should be available for each patient.

Burs

Tooth decay (dental caries) is caused by bacteria (page 60), so it is important that burs for cutting cavities are sterile and, after use, are cleaned and sterilised before being used again.

3-in-1 Tips

On modern dental units the tip of the 3-in-1 syringe can be removed and replaced with a sterile one for the next patient.

Saliva ejectors and suction tips

Plastic types are mainly disposable and must be discarded after use; some are autoclavable. Metal types can be sterilised by heat, ensuring that no debris is trapped on the inner surface before sterilising.

Work surfaces

These should be wiped over between every patient, as well as chair controls, light controls, head rest and bracket table. These are all areas which may become contaminated by saliva and blood. Various recommended cleansers for hard surface are available from dental supply companies.

Particular duties in the surgery
Lay-ups of instruments for specific procedures

Details of relevant instruments to be laid out for particular procedures, in addition to mouth mirror, college tweezers, and straight probe (and the patient's record), will be found on the following pages:

Instructions to patients

Often the DSA is required to assist in the administration of anaesthetics to patients and to give instructions to patients who are about to undergo or who have undergone certain procedures.

Details of assisting, and instructing patients, are given on the following pages:

Dental record charts

Various types of chart are available to enable the dental status of a patient to be recorded graphically. It is essential for the DSA to become familiar with charts in common use, so as to record information on them rapidly and accurately, and to interpret information already recorded.

The complete dentition of an adult normally consists of thirty-two permanent teeth, sixteen in each jaw, eight on each side (or 'quadrant') of the jaw: two incisors (central and lateral), one canine, two premolars (sometimes called 'bi-cuspids') and three molars (the third molars are the 'wisdom teeth'). The natural complement of teeth in a few patients may be less than thirty-two or more.

Children have primary (deciduous or 'milk') teeth, which are replaced by permanent teeth are growth progresses. The deciduous dentition consists of twenty teeth, ten in each jaw, five on each side. They are grouped as follows: two incisors, one canine, and two molars in each half of each jaw. For

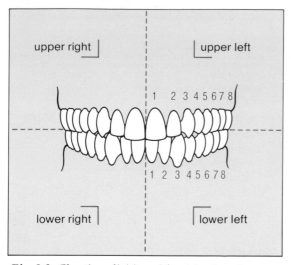

Fig. 1.2 Charting: division of dentition into four quadrants.

descriptions of individual teeth, see Chapter 3.

For charting purposes teeth can be referred to as being 'upper' or 'lower' and 'left' or 'right' (meaning the patient's left or right). In addition, as shown in Figs 1.2 and Figs. 3.1a & b, teeth may be numbered backwards from the front midline. Thus a complete permanent dentition may be written as:

Front Midline
⇩

Patient's   8 7 6 5 4 3 2 1 | 1 2 3 4 5 6 7 8   Patient's
right   8 7 6 5 4 3 2 1 | 1 2 3 4 5 6 7 8   left

The horizontal and vertical lines together are called a 'grid'. Deciduous teeth may be referred to by letter similarly:

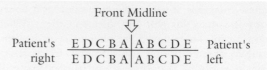

A short form of this notation can be used when referring to particular teeth. For example, a permanent upper left lateral incisor (upper left 2) would be written as $\underline{2}$, and a deciduous lower right second molar (lower right E) would be written as $\overline{E}$. Thus teeth below the horizontal line are 'lower teeth', and teeth written to the left of the vertical line (as you look at it) are actually to the patient's right, and so on. With practice, this system rapidly becomes familiar.

A short-hand way of indicating what teeth a patient has is to write them on a simple grid, leaving spaces for apparently absent teeth (they may have been removed, or may be unformed, or unerupted), and writing x if only the root of a tooth remains.

Here for example is the dentition of an 11 year old:

6 E 4 C 2 1 | 1 2 C E 6 7
7 6 4 3 2 1 | 1 2 3 4 5 7

(Ages at which teeth erupt are given in Fig. 7.1 and Fig. 7.2).

To indicate, for example, upper right 4, some dentists write UR4, and use similar lettering to

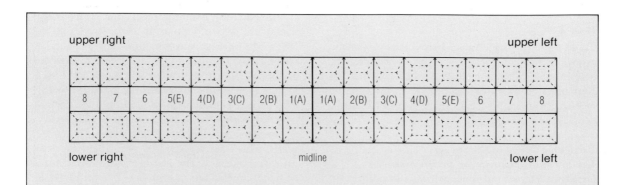

Fig. 1.3 A dental chart grid used by the British National Health Service.

denote the other quadrants (i.e. UL, LR, LL).

You should also familiarise yourself with another system of notation which given each tooth a *two-digit code*. The *second* digit of each code refers to the *tooth*, using the scheme for permanent teeth mentioned earlier. The *first* digit of each code indicates the *quadrant* in which the tooth is found. When the first digit of the code is 1, the tooth is in the upper right quadrant, 2 denotes the upper left quadrant, 3 lower left, and 4 lower right, moving clockwise round the quadrants. The above system refers to *permanent* teeth. Thus an upper right permanent canine (3|) would be referred to a 'tooth 13' (spoken as "one-three", not "thirteen"), and a lower left wisdom tooth (|8) as 'tooth 38' (spoken as "three-eight", not "thirty-eight").

If a *decidious* tooth is to be referred to, the *first* of the two digits is 5 if the tooth is in the upper right quadrant, 6 if upper left, 7 if lower left and 8 if lower right. And the 'deciduous letters' (A, B, C, D, E) become 1, 2, 3, 4, 5. Thus a lower right deciduous canine (C|) would be 'tooth 83' (spoken as "eight-three", not "eighty-three").

A further method of notation for permanent teeth is as follows:

Front Midline
⇩

| 1 | 2 | 3 | 4 | 5 | 6 | 7 | 8 | 9 | 10 | 11 | 12 | 13 | 14 | 15 | 16 |
| 32 | 31 | 30 | 29 | 28 | 27 | 26 | 25 | 24 | 23 | 22 | 21 | 20 | 19 | 18 | 17 |

Deciduous teeth are referred to by letter A–T in the same clockwise pattern:

| A | B | C | D | E | F | G | H | I | J |
| T | S | R | Q | P | O | N | M | L | K |

If all this seems confusing, take heart from the fact that where you work, you will only use one method of notation, not a mixture!

Many dentists use charts based on the above methods of notation on which they record fuller details about the teeth (e.g. fillings present or needed). Figure 1.3 shows a British Chart in which the teeth are numbered as in the first system described above, and a completed charting and descriptive terms are given in Figs 1.4a and 1.4b. Further details about the types of fillings referred to are given on pages 62–63.

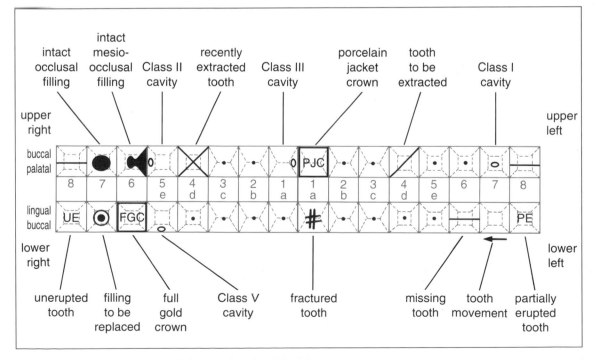

Fig. 1.4a *Sample of a completed charting based on Fig. 1.3.*

Occlusal	–	chewing surface of posterior teeth
Incisal	–	biting surface of anterior teeth
Mesial	–	towards the mid-line
Distal	–	away from the mid-line
Labial	–	towards the lips (incisors and canines)
Buccal	–	towards the cheeks (premolars and molars)
Lingual	–	towards the tongue in the mandible
Palatal	–	towards the palate
Cervical	–	around the neck of the tooth.

Fig. 1.4b List of descriptive terms used in dentistry, as in charting (Fig. 1.4a).

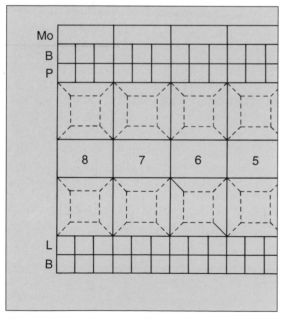

Fig. 1.5 Part of a dental chart with spaces in which to record periodontal pocket depths at six points around each tooth. B = buccal; P = palatal; L = lingual; Mo = mobility (page 107). Several variants of this type of chart exist, some combined with the type shown in Fig. 9.21. Some of the charts include spaces for recording gingival recession.

Figure 1.5 shows how such a chart may be extended to record pocket depths in 'gum disease' (page 105). An alternative to this is shown in Fig 9.21. The 'CPITN' or 'BPE' system of recording 'gum disease' in a mouth is shown in Fig. 9.19.

The wearing of dentures is often recorded, such as, for example, P/– (meaning an upper partial denture but no lower denture) and F/P (meaning an upper full or complete denture, with no natural teeth remaining, and a lower partial denture).

X-ray films (radiographs)

X-rays cannot be seen. They are a form of radiation able to affect photographic film in a way similar to light after passing to a varying extent through objects of different density, such as teeth and bone. The image produced, once developed, is rather like a shadow graph, with the hardest materials (such as tooth enamel or metal fillings) appearing white, and less hard materials appearing darker. Comparing these varying densities on an X-ray film can help the dentist in diagnosis. Once the image on the film can be seen, it is called a radiograph.

Although very useful in diagnosis, X-rays can also be dangerous. To minimise the risks, the following precautions are essential:

1. *Protection of the patient.* Female patients of child-bearing years should be asked if they might be pregnant. Because of risk to the fetus, pregnant patients should not be X-rayed. During X-rays all patients should wear a lead apron which covers the thyroid gland in the neck and extends to cover the reproductive organs. As radiation has a cumulative effect on the body, patients must be asked when they last had any X-ray films taken and whether they have received any radiation treatment in the past. Unnecessary X-ray films are to be avoided, which means that care is needed when taking and developing X-ray films.

2. *Protection of staff.* Operators should wear lead aprons and stand 1.5 metres away from the X-ray machine head, directly behind the direction of the X-ray beam, or preferably behind a lead screen. Wearing an X-ray monitoring badge (Fig 1.6) is advisable. Your machine must be switched off when not in use, and it should be checked professionally every year.

> Operators must NEVER, under any circumstances, hold X-ray films inside or outside a patient's mouth during exposure to the X-ray beam.

Types of X-ray film
X-Ray films used in dentistry are of two types:

• Intra-oral (used inside the patient's mouth)
• Extra-oral (used outside the patient's mouth)

Examples of each type are given below:

Intra-oral films	View
Periapical	One or two teeth from crown to root tip (apex) and associated bone, and diseases of these structures, root fragments, unerupted teeth, and other pathology. Essential for root canal therapy. Useful for periodontal diagnosis.
Bite-wing (Fig 1.7)	Upper and lower molar and premolar teeth in occlusion. Shows the contact point between the teeth, caries at these sites and elsewhere, bone crests and the top of the roots. If the long axis of the film is mounted vertically, more of the root can be seen.
Occlusal (large packet, held along the biting surface of the teeth)	Show the arch of the teeth and structures to the 'sides' of the teeth, such as unerupted teeth in the palate and a stone in a salivary duct.

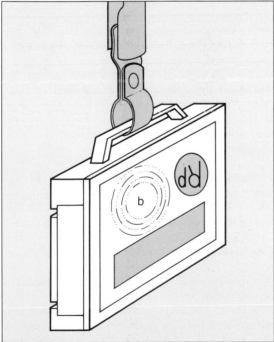

Fig. 1.6 X-ray monitoring badge in use in the UK carrying an X-ray film wrapped in foil. The wearer's name, printed on the foil, is visible through the rectangular window in the plastic cover. The letters RP are visible through the round window. The side of the badge which faces towards the source of X-rays also has a prominent bulge (b).

Extra-oral film

Orthopantomograph (OPT or OPG)	Taken in special machines, and show the entire jaws and teeth, and temporo-mandibular joints. A useful basic assessment film.
Lateral oblique film	For buried lower wisdom teeth.
Lateral skull cephalometry	For orthodontic assessment of skull, lower jaw, erupted and unerupted teeth.

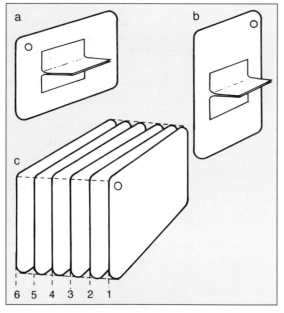

Fig. 1.7 Standard periapical X-ray film packets showing the raised dot or 'blip' which faces towards the X-ray machine in use. 'Bite-wing tabs' are also shown, positioned to obtain (a) horizontal bite-wing films, and (b) vertical bite-wing films. (c) is an 'exploded' view to show the contents of such a packet: 1 - pebbled plastic front cover with raised dot; 2 - black paper; 3 - X-ray film; 4 - lead film (to stop further progress of X-rays); 5 - foil with herring-bone pattern; 6 - smooth plastic back cover with tab for opening packet.

Intra-oral films are placed with a dot or blip towards the tube. (The developed film also has a similar blip to show the direction from which it should be viewed.) Extra-oral films are placed in metal 'intensifying screens' to reduce the radiation needed to expose them. Other extra-oral films are available, and any type may sometimes be needed to assess disease in adjacent structures (e.g. the sinuses) and jaw fractures.

Processing of X-ray films
If done in a photographic darkroom, this involves the following sequence:

1. The darkroom door is locked, the safelight is switched on, and the main light is switched off.

2. Films are arranged on hangers according to a scheme which allows them to be accurately identified after developing.

3. Film packets are unwrapped and replaced on the hangers.

4. The films on the hanger are placed in freshly prepared developer for the recommended time and at the correct temperature.

5. The developed films are washed in water.

6. The films are transferred to fresh fixer solution for the recommended time and at the correct temperature.

7. Films are washed thoroughly in running tap water.

8. The films are dried, identified (see 2 above) and dated, viewed by the dentist, and filed in the patient's notes.

The above procedure (1 – 7) has been superseded in many practices by automatic processors.

A method of taking dental radiographs without the use of X-ray film (radiovisiography) is coming into use; doses of radiation are much lower than existing methods, and delays in processing are avoided.

Health and safety
All dental establishments, staff and patients are covered by the provisions of the Health and Safety at Work Act. This seeks to protect patients and staff by

making them aware of the hazards in the work place and encourage them to find the best way of ensuring the work place is a safe place for all.

The practice manager should be informed immediately of any faults which may be hazardous to patients or staff (e.g. in electrical equipment, seating, flooring, or stairs).

Waiting areas

Flooring and lighting should be in good condition, especially on stairs. Seating should be safe for all patients. All wiring from telephones, heaters, fish tanks, etc., should be positioned safely. Toys should be checked for sharp edges, and any bits which a small child could swallow removed; broken toys should be discarded.

Treatment areas

As for *Waiting areas*. Also chemicals, autoclaves, sharps, etc., should be out of the reach of patients to prevent accidental burns, scalds or other injury.

Laboratories

As other areas, taking extreme care with flammable liquids, bunsen burners, chemicals, etc.

Fire drills

Staff should practise using fire escapes, and note the location and use of fire extinguishers.

Drugs

The DSA needs to be familiar with the strict regulations which apply whenever drugs are kept in a dental surgery for prescribing to patients.

Controlled and other drugs need to be kept in a locked and fixed container, and some require refrigeration. Only the minimum required routinely should be kept. Prescription pads also need to be kept securely.

Drugs can only be ordered and prescribed by the dentist. Records need to be kept for 11 years concerning:

- the quantity, source, and date of each supply

- full details of each prescription to individual patients

Drugs should not be taken out of the manufacturer's original packs, and any warnings and instructions should not be removed. Childproof containers should be used for drugs not supplied pre-packed. "Accountable" drugs should be returned to the pharmacy if out of date, but other drugs should be disposed of down the toilet, not put in waste bags.

Accidents

Each dental practice should have an accident book in which all accidents to staff or patients are recorded.

- Accidents in the surgery include injuries from sharp (possibly contaminated) instruments.

Procedure for injuries caused by needles or sharp instruments:

Identify instrument if possible, and inform senior members of staff.

Squeeze the wound to encourage bleeding and hold under running water.

Apply antiseptic to area and cover with dry dressing.

Observe injury site for infection - seek medical advice.

Check the medical history of the patient on whom the instrument was used for evidence of hepatitis B.

Record the incident in the accident book.

The accident book must be filled in for every accident, however trivial, affecting patients or staff.

Control of substances hazardous to health (C.O.S.H.H)

All substances which can be potentially harmful come under the strict regulations of C.O.S.H.H. In the dental surgery we use a great number of substances which can be harmful, for example:
Waste amalgam
Mercury
Chemical sterilising solutions
Flammable substances/liquids

Your surgery should have a copy of the C.O.S.H.H regulations. The following guidelines may be helpful:

Chemical sterilising solutions

The container should have a lid to prevent any vapours escaping. Wear gloves, mask and protective eye wear when handling. Any instruments placed in these solutions must be completely immersed for 8 hours to ensure sterilisation, and then rinsed thoroughly with distilled water prior to use. People who suffer from asthma or other respiratory disorders may find their condition is affected.

Flammable Liquids (e.g. cold-cure acrylic)
Store away from sunlight and other forms of heat. Use in a well ventilated area away from bunsen burners, etc.

Procedures for dealing with waste amalgam and mercury spillage are described on page 62.

• Non-clinical role of the DSA

Non-clinical duties are usually carried out by the receptionist who may also be a qualified DSA. A range of possible duties are as follows:

- Greet all patients with a smile and with a courteous manner.

- Arrange appointments and ensure that all re-call appointments are sent.

- File patients' notes, forms and X-ray films in the correct file, and provide the correct notes for the Dental Surgeon as required.

- Answer the telephone promptly and deal with callers efficiently and in a professional way.

- Encourage high standards of health and safety in all areas used by patients and staff.

- Order stock from suppliers.

- Communicate with the dental laboratories regarding collection and delivery procedures.

- Arrange with Company Representatives the most appropriate time to visit or telephone the Dental Surgeon.

- Be responsible for receiving payments by patients, issuing change and receipts correctly.

- Inform the Dental Surgeon, DSA, or Hygienist when patients arrive for treatment or cancel.

- Operate the computer, and process patients' forms for payment.

USEFUL ADDRESSES

The Secretary
Examining Board (EBDSA)
DSA House
29 London Street
Fleetwood
Lancs, FY7 6JY
Telephone: 0253 778417

The same address should be used for information regarding the Association of British DSAs (Secretary ABDSA), and also for details on the Voluntary National Register for DSAs (Registrar).

British Dental Hygienists Association
64 Wimpole Street
London, W1M 8AL
Telephone: 071 935 0875

General Dental Council
37 Wimpole Street
London, W1M 8DQ
Telephone 071-486 2171

The School of Dentistry
Grosvenor Road
Belfast
Northern Ireland, BT12 6BP

The Dental School
St. Chad's Queensway
Birmingham, B4 6NN

The Dental School
Lower Maudlin Street
Bristol, BS1 2LY

The Dental School
Park Place
Dundee, DD1 4HN

Eastman Dental Hospital
Gray's Inn Road
London, WC1X 8LD

The School of Dental Surgery
Chambers Street
Edinburgh, EH1 1JA

The Dental School
378 Sauchiehall Street
Glasgow, G2 3JZ

*Dental School of the United Medical
and Dental Schools of Guy's and
St. Thomas's Hospitals
London Bridge
London, SE1 9RT*

*King's College School of Medicine and Dentistry
Denmark Hill
London, SE5 8RX*

*The Dental School and Hospital
Clarendon Way
Leeds, LS2 9LU*

*The School of Dental Surgery
Pembroke Place
PO Box 147
Liverpool, L3 5PS*

*The London Hospital Medical College
Dental School
Turner Street
London, E1 2AD*

*The Turner Dental School
Higher Cambridge Street
Manchester, M15 6FH*

*The Dental School
Newcastle-upon-Tyne Dental Hospital
Richardson Road
Newcastle-upon-Tyne, NE2 4AZ*

*University of Wales College of Medicine
Dental School
Heath Park
Cardiff, CF4 4XY*

*The School of Clinical Dentistry
Charles Clifford Dental Hospital
Wellesley Road
Sheffield, S10 2SZ*

When you write for personal advice about a course, you should give full details of your education to date and your age.

2. General Anatomy and Physiology

Human anatomy studies how the body is built, and physiology how the various parts of the body function. Anatomical descriptions often use special terms to describe the relationships between structures:

Superior: Above	Lateral: Towards the outside
Inferior: Below	Medial: Towards the inside

LIVING ORGANISMS

Seven basic functions characterise living organisms:

1. Breathing: Intake of oxygen from the air to be used for processing into energy. The chemical processes involved are termed 'respiration'.

2. Feeding: Intake of food to be used as fuel for energy, heat, growth and repair.

3. Excretion: The elimination of unwanted waste products from the body. For example, carbon dioxide is a waste product of respiration, eliminated from the lungs to the air during breathing. Food waste is eliminated from the body as faeces. Water-soluble waste products are eliminated via the kidneys as urine.

4. Reproduction.

5. Growth.

6. Movement.

7. Irritability: The ability of a living creature to respond to its environment.

CELLS

The human body and all living organisms are composed of cells. A cell is the smallest unit of the body which can exist by itself, and has a highly complex microscopic structure and chemical make-up. Typically, a cell (Fig. 2.1) is composed of a jelly-like material called 'cytoplasm', consisting of protein, small amounts of fat, sugars (carbohydrates), vitamins and salts (such as sodium chloride, potassium chloride and sodium bicarbonate) dissolved in water. Water occupies approximately seventy percent of the volume of each cell. The cytoplasm performs the essential biochemical functions to maintain the cell as a living unity. This is called 'cell metabolism'.

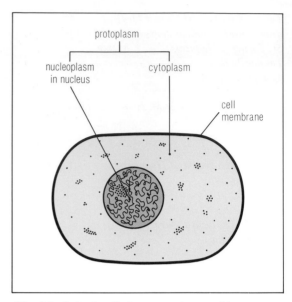

Fig. 2.1 *A single cell of an organism, and its components.*

Embedded in the cytoplasm is the 'nucleus' which is a highly specialised structure enclosed by the nuclear membrane. The nucleus controls all functions of the cell and contains the genetic material, chromosomes, which carry hereditary information from one generation of cells to the next. This information is carried by a complex and very important material called 'deoxyribonucleic acid' (DNA). The jelly-like material in the nucleus is called 'nucleoplasm'. The combination of cytoplasm and nucleoplasm is termed 'protoplasm'.

The entire animal cell is covered by a flexible cell membrane which allows nutrients to penetrate and waste products to pass out. The human body is built up of millions of cells, each able to perform the seven vital functions which are characteristic of life. Cells performing similar functions are grouped together and form 'tissues', groups of tissues form 'organs', and organs form 'systems'. The different systems of the body form the organism (Fig. 2.2).

Cell types

Although the body is composed of millions of individual cells, there are only four different basic cell types to be found: epithelial, connective, muscle and nerve. Groups of these cells form tissues named accordingly.

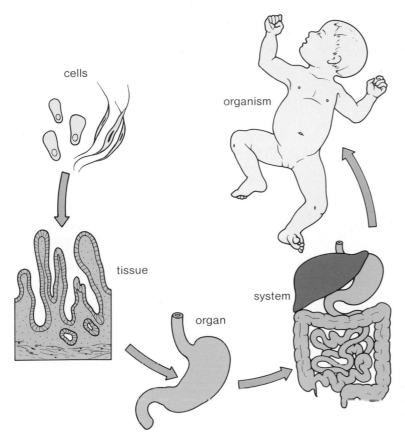

Fig. 2.2 *Development of the human organism: from cells to tissues, tissues to organs, organs to a complete system.*

Epithelial tissue

Epithelial tissue consists of a sheet-like layer of cells which cover a free surface, for example, the skin of the outer body surface, the lining of the mouth (oral cavity) and the intestines, nasal and airway passages, the lining of the lumen of blood vessels, and the urinary tubular system. The intercellular cement, binding one cell to its neighbour, is of minimal thickness. In addition, some collections of epithelial cells form glandular tissue which manufactures substances required by the body; for example, the salivary glands secrete saliva which lubricates and protects the oral cavity. The epithelial lining of the oral cavity is, therefore, normally moistened with saliva. A moist epithelium is termed 'mucous membrane' or 'mucosa'.

Connective tissue

This is never found on a free surface, except in disease or injury. It is composed of cells and an intercellular cement but, unlike epithelial tissues, the intercellular material is a major component of the tissue and gives it its physical characteristics. For example, blood is a kind of connective tissue where the intercellular cement is a fluid and the cells are blood cells. This arrangement allows the free-flowing movement of blood. On the other hand, cartilage has a more plastic type of intercellular cement and is found where rigidity and flexibility are required.

Loose connective tissue is found in the body as a type of 'packing' material between its various components and organs. The jelly-like intercellular cement gives the physical properties of flexibility and support.

Bone has an intercellular cement rich in calcium salts, making it very rigid and strong, for support and protection of the body. Adipose tissue is responsible for fat storage, and is found just beneath the skin.

Muscle tissue

Muscle cells are special in that they have the ability to alter their shape by contraction, hence muscles are responsible for movement. Three types of muscle tissue exist:

Skeletal, responsible for bodily movements such as bending, walking and running. These movements are under voluntary control; that is to say, they may be started or stopped at will.

Smooth, responsible for movement of the internal organs of the body such as the stomach, bowels, gall bladder, hair follicles and blood vessels. These movements are controlled automatically and are beyond voluntary control (i.e. autonomic).

Cardiac, found exclusively in the heart. This muscle is also under involuntary (autonomic) control but, unlike the other types of muscle, it has the ability to contract in more than one direction at a time.

Nerve tissue

Nerve cells are specially modified to conduct electrical impulses, thus forming the 'communications' system of the body.

ORGANS AND SYSTEMS

An organ is a functioning part of the body which contains all four cells types. The organs of the body are collected together as systems. There are ten different systems within the body. It is very important to realise that each system does not work independently of the others, but that all systems work together as one functional unit, namely, the human body. The body systems are:

1. Integumentary: The protective covering of the body, forming an effective barrier to infection and water loss, as well as perception of sensations such as temperature, pain and touch. The skin also plays an important part in the regulation of body temperature, the average normal being 37°C. If the body is overheated (due to a high external temperature or as a result of infection and fever), then blood supply to the skin is increased and sweating occurs in an attempt to reduce the body temperature back to normal. Conversely, the blood vessels in the skin contract and reduce the blood supply in an attempt to conserve heat within the body when cold.

2. Skeletal: The bony framework of the body, giving support and protection to structures such as the brain, heart and lungs. The joints between bones enable movement. Bone also acts as a calcium store.

3. Muscular: The system of muscles, together with the skeletal framework, enabling movement to take place.

4. Cardiovascular: The heart and system of vessels (arteries and veins), distributing blood to all parts of the body. The lymphatic system of vessels forms an alternative route for the absorption of tissue fluid and its return to the blood.

5. Alimentary (Digestive): The food pathways, processing ingested food so that essential nutrients may be extracted and used.

6. Respiratory: The lungs and air passages, conducting oxygen in and carbon dioxide (waste gas) out.

7. Urinary: The kidneys and bladder, responsible for eliminating excess water and water-soluble waste products from the body.

8. Reproductive (Genital): The system responsible for reproduction.

9. Endocrine: Glands, producing hormones which enter directly, and circulate in, the bloodstream to regulate important chemical processes of the body. Examples are the thyroid gland which controls the rate at which the body uses energy, and the pituitary gland which controls many functions including normal growth.

10. Nervous: The brain and all nerves, forming the mechanism that governs movement (motor function) and perception of light, sound, touch, temperature, smell and pain (sensory function). The brain also controls involuntary functions, such as contraction and movement of the intestines.

Cells in the body require oxygen, which is used in all systems to produce energy from the cell's stores of materials, such as carbohydrates (sugars), derived from food. Waste products from these chemical reactions are harmful to the body if allowed to accumulate to any degree, and have to be eliminated.

The respiratory and cardiovascular systems are responsible for conveying oxygen to all cells. Blood carries the carbohydrates and other nutrients extracted from ingested food by the digestive system. Waste products are collected from the cells into the blood, and the cardiovascular system delivers water-soluble waste to the kidneys for elimination through the urinary tract; carbon dioxide gas is eliminated through the lungs. Figure 2.3 shows the interrelationships of these systems.

CARDIOVASCULAR SYSTEM

The cardiovascular system consists of the heart and the blood vessels which circulate and distribute blood to all parts of the body. Circulation is performed by the pumping action of the heart. The vessels which carry blood away from the heart to the body cells are known as arteries, and those which collect blood from the cells and return it to the heart are known as

veins. The change from artery to vein occurs at capillaries and exchanges between blood and cells occur across the delicate capillary walls.

The heart

The heart lies in the chest cavity, slightly towards the left side. It is protected by the rib cage and the breast bone (sternum), which also protect the lungs. The heart consists of four chambers, two on the left and two on the right. The chambers on the left are completely separated from those on the right by a dense muscle wall called 'septum'. The two chambers on each side communicate with each other. However, blood flows in one direction only, from one chamber to the other. A system of valves separates the two chambers on each side to ensure correct flow (Fig. 2.4).

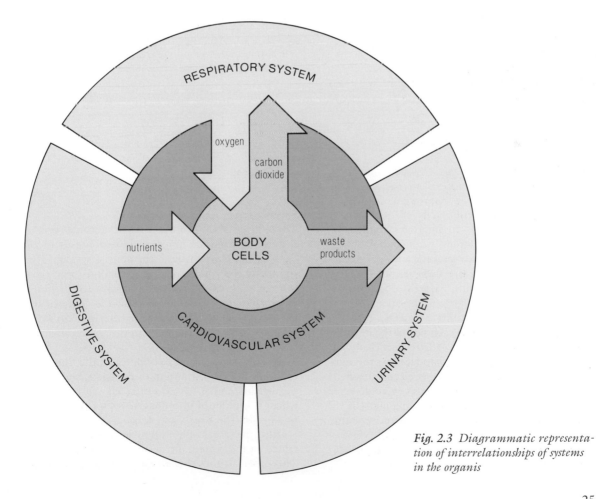

Fig. 2.3 Diagrammatic representation of interrelationships of systems in the organis

25

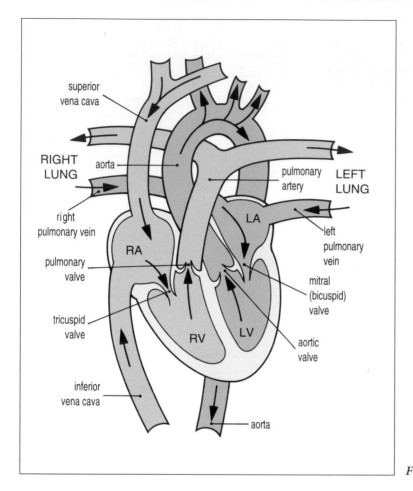

superior
vena cava

RIGHT
LUNG

aorta

pulmonary
artery

LEFT
LUNG

right
pulmonary vein

LA

left
pulmonary
vein

RA

pulmonary
valve

mitral
(bicuspid)
valve

tricuspid
valve

RV

LV

aortic
valve

inferior
vena cava

aorta

Fig. 2.4   *The heart and great vessels.*

Diseases, such as rheumatic fever, may damage the valves, which leads to improper circulation. Damage may also occur as a congenital defect. Patients with a history of rheumatic fever or congenital heart disease are at risk from serious bacterial heart infection (sub-acute bacterial endocarditis) from some dental procedures. Such patients require antibiotic cover to prevent this (page 108).

The upper chambers on each side of the heart are called 'atria', the lower are called 'ventricles'. The pumping action of the heart (produced by the muscle walls contracting) results from electrical activity within the heart muscle itself. This can be detected by the use of sensitive electronic equipment at the surface of the body. Electrodes are placed on arms, legs, and chest wall and connected to an 'electrocardiograph', and a printed record of the heart's electrical activity is produced (ECG; Fig. 2.5).

Circulation

The left side of the heart receives oxygenated (bright red) blood from the lungs, and distributes it to all parts of the body through the arterial system. The right side receives deoxygenated blood (blue-red) from all parts of the body and sends it to the lungs to be reoxygenated. This is known as 'pulmonary circulation'. The left side of the heart distributes blood to the rest of the body in the 'systemic circulation' (Fig. 2.6).

Freshly oxygenated blood from the lungs is received into the left atrium of the heart, and passes through the mitral valve into the left ventricle, from where it is pumped into the arteries for distribution to all cells. The large vessel leaving the left ventricle is called the 'aorta'. Blood flow in the aorta is maintained in the correct direction by the aortic valves. The other arteries branch from the aorta and are

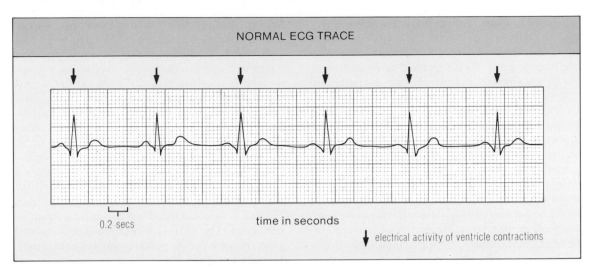

Fig. 2..5 A normal cardiographic trace. ECGs are printed records of the heart's electrical activity.

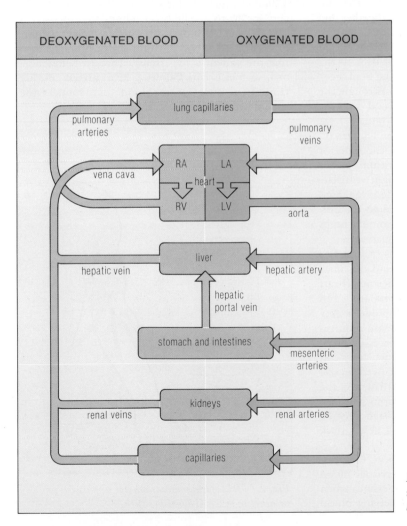

Fig. 2.6 Diagrammatic representation of the human blood circulation.

distributed to all parts of the body. The first branches of the aorta are in the coronary arteries, which supply the heart muscle itself. Coronary artery disease leads to poor blood supply of the heart muscle which, as a result, cannot perform its pumping action correctly. Patients suffering from this condition experience severe chest pain (angina) as soon as they attempt any exertion.

Each heartbeat produces an injection of blood into the aorta and the subsequent arteries. The arteries which are close to the skin (for example, the radial artery on the inner surface of the wrist), can be felt to pulsate in response to each heart contraction. The patient's radial pulse will, therefore, give direct information regarding the rate and strength of the heart contraction.

The final small arteries form thin capillaries, where exchange of oxygen as well as of nutritional and waste products occurs within the cells. The capillaries unite to form veins which join together and form increasingly larger vessels (veins) returning to the heart. Two major veins collect venous blood from all parts of the body and carry it back to the right atrium of the heart. Blood from the head, neck and upper part of the trunk returns through the superior vena cava (Fig. 2.4), whilst blood from the lower limbs, lower trunk and abdominal areas returns through the inferior vena cava. The deoxygenated (venous) blood, arriving via the superior and inferior vena cava to the right atrium, passes through the tricuspid valve into the right ventricle. Each heart contraction expels the deoxygenated blood to the right and left lungs through the pulmonary arteries. Reoxygenated blood from the lungs returns to the heart through the pulmonary vein.

Disease of the heart or blood vessels may lead to high blood pressure (hypertension), and the heart muscle may eventually fail to pump efficiently (heart failure). To prevent this, such patients are given tablets to control their elevated blood pressure. Any patient with heart or circulatory disease requires careful dental treatment and should never be given an out-patient general anaesthetic, as circulatory collapse and death may easily ensue. If the heart muscle suddenly becomes unable to pump efficiently, the patient will become pale, sweaty, anxious and may collapse. This a 'heart attack'. Surgery staff must be prepared to manage a patient having a heart attack (see page 155).

At the peak of ventricular contraction, the pressure in the arterial system is greatest (systolic blood pressure). It is least (diastolic blood pressure) when the ventricles are totally relaxed, receiving blood

from the left auricle and awaiting the next contraction. Arterial blood pressure is measured by placing an inflatable cuff around the upper arm of a patient, linked to a sphygmomanometer containing a gauge or tube of mercury (Fig. 2.7). Blood pressure is expressed as equivalent to the pressure exerted by a vertical column of mercury measured in millimetres. The systolic blood pressure is determined by inflating the cuff until the pressure stops the pulse felt at the wrist. This is verified by listening with a stethoscope for the loss of the pulse sound in the main arteries below the cuff in the bend of the elbow (antecubital fossa). The mercury gauge is then read. The cuff is slowly deflated and the pulse is heard to start again. The diastolic blood pressure is reached when the sound of the pulse can no longer be heard. The mercury gauge is read again.

Normal blood pressure is approximately 100–120mm of mercury for systolic, 70–80mm of mercury for diastolic. The two readings are expressed as 100/70 (said 100 over 70). Such a patient is 'normotensive'. A blood pressure above normal shows that the patient is hypertensive, whilst below normal, such as occurs following heart attacks, during fainting or after severe blood loss, renders the patient hypotensive.

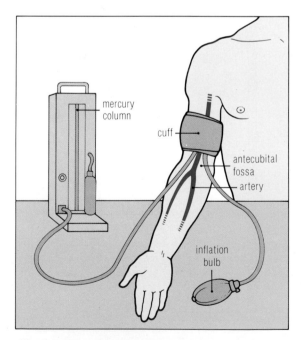

Fig. 2.7 *The sphyngmomanometer apparatus for measuring arterial blood pressure.*

THE LYMPHATIC SYSTEM

This system of vessels, similar in structure to veins, runs throughout the body and helps regulate the fluid balance of the body. The vessels contain a pale yellow fluid (lymph) in which lymphocytes circulate. Lymphocytes circulate in the lymph and blood in almost equal numbers. Lymph vessels drain into the venous side of the blood circulation system. At intervals along the course of the vessels there are collections of lymphoid tissue called 'nodes' which are the source of lymphocytes. Lymphocytes and nodes act to protect the body against spread of infection. The lymph system, including the nodes, may also become involved in the spread of cancer. The head and neck regions of the body are particularly rich in lymph nodes and these are important because if they become enlarged or tender (or both), this may indicate the presence of disease in the region drained by the vessels serving the affected nodes.

RESPIRATORY SYSTEM

Respiration consists of two phases:

Inhaling and exhaling air. This is known as breathing or external respiration.

The chemical processes taking place between the cells of the body and bloodstream, whereby oxygen and carbon dioxide are exchanged (internal respiration). The respiratory system is depicted in Fig. 2.8.

Breathing

Air enters the respiratory system through the nose or mouth (inspiration). The internal surface of the nasal cavity has a large surface areas created by small projections or bone (turbinate bones) from the lateral walls of the nasal cavity. The internal surface is covered by a moist epithelium (nasal mucosa) which ensures that the inhaled air is humid. The mucous

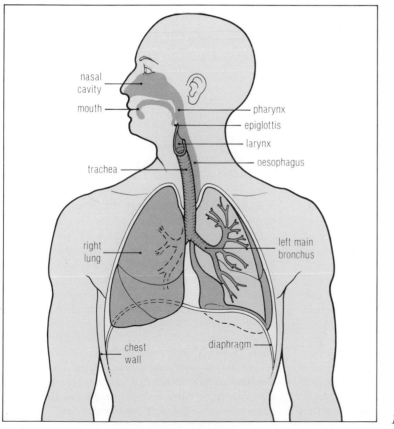

Fig. 2.8 The respiratory system.

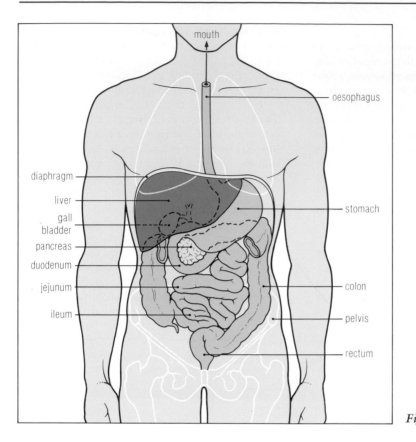

Fig. 2.9 The alimentary system.

membrane is also richly supplied with blood vessels carrying warm blood close to the surface. The inspired air is thereby also warmed. It then passes through the larynx (in the throat) which contains the vocal chords responsible for creating the sounds of speech. Below the larynx there is a hollow tube, the trachea, which runs into the chest. The lumen of the trachea is prevented from collapsing by rings of cartilage in its walls. The trachea ends in the chest by dividing into two main branches, the bronchi, one bronchus serving each lung. The lungs and heart lie in the chest, protected from injury by the rib cage and sternum.

Muscles between the ribs move them upwards and downwards, causing air to enter and be expelled from the lungs. A sheet of muscle, called the 'diaphragm' forms the floor of the chest cavity and separates the contents of the chest from the contents of the abdomen. Downward movement of the diaphragm and upward movement of the ribs aids inspiration. When the act of inspiration is complete, the upward movement of the diaphragm and downward movement of the ribs causes air to be driven from the lungs back through the airway and thence to the atmosphere (expiration). This anatomical pathway is exclusively reserved for air, and obstruction of the airway occurs if food or other material enters the passage. Normally, in consciousness, any such obstruction is expelled by automatic coughing. During general anaesthesia when consciousness is lost, these protective reflexes are also lost, and it is the anaesthetist's responsibility not only to administer the anaesthetic, but also to ensure safety of the patient's airway until consciousness returns.

Inhaled air ultimately enters the fine structure of the lung called 'air-sacs', which are of a single cell thickness surrounded by fine blood capillaries. Here, gases are exchanged with the bloodstream.

ALIMENTARY SYSTEM

This system (Fig. 2.9) processes food and extracts from it useful nutrients required by the body's cells. Nutrients are carried from the digestive tract to the cells through the bloodstream. The process of digestion begins with mastication of food into small digestible particles. During this process, saliva is stimulated to flow into the mouth and mix with food, making it easily swallowed to pass through the oesophagus into the stomach. The act of swallowing is called 'deglutition'.

At the onset of swallowing, food is forced from the mouth into the oesophagus across the top of the entrance the airway. The soft palate rises and seals the entrance at the back of the nose. A cartilaginous flap, called the 'epiglottis', covers the airway entrance as food passes towards the oesophagus. Once the ball of food in paste form (bolus) enters the oesophagus, the muscular walls of the oesophagus contract in a wave-like fashion ('peristalsis') and drive the bolus downwards, into the stomach.

The stomach lies just below the diaphragm. It has a muscular wall and a mucous membrane lining containing glands which secrete acid and enzymes. The acid kills many types of bacteria (thus protecting the body from harmful bacterial invasion), and also creates the correct conditions for special chemicals (gastric enzymes) to break down the food into its component parts. Food remains in the stomach for about four hours, during which time it is mixed with the enzymes by contraction and relaxation of the muscular walls of the stomach. On leaving the stomach, the partly digested food enters the duodenum which has its own glandular mucosa. Duodenal secretions neutralise the acidic stomach contents and add further enzymes which continue the process of digestion. The pancreas secretes its digestive enzymes, delivered into the duodenum by the pancreatic duct (Fig. 2.10).

By further peristaltic movements of the muscular walls which extend throughout the digestive tube (alimentary canal), food enters the coiled small intestine (approximately six metres in length), where digestion is complete. The blood capillaries in the mucosal lining of the intestinal wall transfer the useful products of digestion to the blood circulation. The

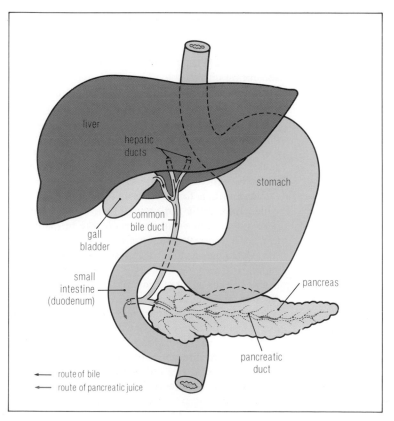

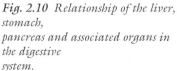

Fig. 2.10 *Relationship of the liver, stomach, pancreas and associated organs in the digestive system.*

remaining bulky waste passes to the large intestine where water is removed into the blood circulation. The semi-solid waste is expelled from the body (defaecation), via the rectum and anus.

The liver

Blood, rich in absorbed nutrients collected from the capillaries in the walls of the intestine, is conveyed to the liver by increasingly larger veins. There the veins break up into another fine capillary bed in association with the cells of the liver. The liver cells store and process many of the nutrients. Several drugs are removed from the blood by the liver at this stage. The capillaries then reform into a large vein which returns blood to the heart via the inferior vena cava. This vein-capillary-vein system forms the hepatic portal system.

The liver also generates essential substances, such as blood proteins (plasma proteins) and bile. Bile is stored in the gall bladder and released into the duodenum where it mixes with the partly digested food. Bile not only acts as a means of ridding the body of bile-soluble waste products, such as some drugs, but is also essential for the processing and absorption of fat into the blood stream. Some essential fat soluble vitamins are absorbed only in the presence of bile.

Obstruction of the normal flow of bile from the liver to the duodenum eventually leads to bile spilling over into the blood circulation, giving the patient's skin and whites of the eyes (sclera) a yellow colour. This is known as jaundice, and can occur after some drug treatments, viral infections such as hepatitis, or stones in the gall bladder which obstruct the bile duct. The latter can also be obstructed by external compression, for example by a cancer of the pancreas. Some blood diseases also cause jaundice, but jaundice nearly always reflects liver problems.

Liver disease and dentistry is discussed on page 59.

Useful products of digestion

These are proteins, carbohydrates, fat, vitamins and minerals. Proteins are largely found in meat, fish, eggs and dairy products such as milk and cheese. They are broken down into their component amino acids which are absorbed directly into the blood from the small intestine. They are then used by the body to build new proteins, the essential component of all cells of the body.

Carbohydrates are sugars that provide energy and are primarily found in sugar, flour and potatoes. The basic component of all sugars is glucose. Digestion of carbohydrates produces glucose units which are absorbed into the blood stream from the small intestine. The circulating level of glucose in the blood has to be maintained very carefully by the body. A hormone produced in the pancreas, insulin, is primarily responsible for keeping blood sugar at normal levels. This is secreted directly into the blood stream. If blood sugar is allowed to rise, then the patient becomes very susceptible to infections, particularly of the mouth and skin. Also, high levels of sugar in the circulating blood cause the kidneys to produce large amounts of urine containing some of the excess glucose. Such a patient is diabetic.

Fats are abundant in dairy products. Their basic unit is a fatty-acid which is produced during their digestion. Bile is necessary for fat absorption into the blood stream. Fat acts as a reserve energy supply and is stored just beneath the skin where, due to its nature, it also acts as a layer of insulation reducing heat loss.

Vitamins are essential compounds for normal function of the body. Only very small amounts are required, but as many vitamins are not stored in the body, a continuous supply from food is necessary. Many different vitamins have been discovered and each is identified by a letter of the alphabet. The most important vitamins for the DSA to know about are B, C, and D. Vitamins B and C are water-soluble. Vitamin D is fat-soluble, and requires bile for its absorption into the blood stream. Jaundiced patients may, therefore, become deficient in vitamin D. Vitamin B consists of a collection of compounds forming an essential part of the chemical processes of all cells. They also play an important role in the formation of blood cells. Deficiency of vitamin B causes a type of anaemia which often presents with soreness of the tongue (glossitis).

Vitamin C is found in fresh fruit and vegetables which have not been overcooked, as heat rapidly destroys it. It plays an important role in many cell functions, especially the formation of connective tissue. Deficiency (scurvy) manifests with fragile blood capillaries and a tendency to bleed, particularly noticeable as severe gum disease with bleeding. Vitamin D is found in meat, fish (especially cod and halibut liver), milk, eggs, and cheese. It plays an extremely important role in calcium absorption into the blood stream from food. It is essential, together with calcium for the normal development and growth of bone and teeth. Vitamin D deficiency (rickets) produces abnormalities in the calcified tissues of the body.

Minerals, or trace elements, are required by the body in very small amounts. Like vitamins, a constant supply from food is essential. Important minerals for the DSA to know about are calcium, phosphorus and iron. Calcium and phosphorus are found in milk, eggs and other dairy products. Iron is the basis of the red blood cell oxygen-carrying pigment called 'haemoglobin'. Iron deficiency causes anaemia, whereby the blood's capacity to carry oxygen is greatly reduced. Oral complications of anaemia are a sore, smooth tongue (glossitis) and soreness of the oral mucosa.

Water

The average 70kg adult person contains approximately forty litres of water. This percentage content is accurately controlled by the body, and for normal function it must not vary greatly. Water is absorbed from the gut. Excess amounts are eliminated via the kidney as urine. Water loss also occurs from the lungs during breathing, by sweating, and in the form of digestive juices. Deprivation of drink or excessive fluid loss rapidly causes improper functioning of the body's cells, and requires urgent treatment.

BLOOD

Blood distributes nutrients to each cell and carries away harmful waste products for safe elimination from the body. The exchange of nutrients and waste occurs with blood capillaries which form a network associated with each cell. Oxygenated blood is carried to the capillaries by arteries, and deoxygenated blood is carried away for the capillaries by veins (see Circulation, pages 26 and 27). An obstruction within the lumen of an artery is called an 'embolus'. The blockage deprives the area supplied by that artery of oxygen and nutrients, and this leads to localised cell death (necrosis). The area of dead tissue is called an 'infarct'. A blockage in a vein (thrombus) causes a similar disruption in the circulation in the area it drains.

The average 70kg adult contains approximately five litres of blood. Blood itself contains three types of cell: red, white and platelets, plus a supporting fluid called plasma. The main function of red cells is to carry oxygen. Each red cell contains an oxygen-carrying pigment called 'haemoglobin', an important constituent of which is the iron obtained from digested food. Oxygenated haemoglobin gives the blood is bright red colour. White cells are responsible for the body's defence against disease, by destroying invading bacteria and viruses. White cells are taken to all parts of the body through blood circulation, and perform this protective function wherever invasion occurs. Platelets play an important role in the prevention of blood loss following injury, by clumping together on site, forming a seal to the damaged vessels whilst formation of a blood clot occurs. Blood plasma is a slightly yellow substance consisting mainly of water plus dissolved proteins (plasma proteins). Some of these (antibodies) are responsible for attacking infective agents. Others form the blood clot to seal a damaged area to prevent blood loss and promote healing. Blood, therefore, performs many important functions in the body, summarised as follows:

1. Transport of oxygen to the body's cells, via haemoglobin in the red cells.

2. Carriage of waste products, such as carbon dioxide, to the lungs.

3. Distribution of ingested nutrients from the digestive tract to the body's cells.

4. The plasma proteins carry hormones to all parts of the body. These hormones have an important regulatory effect upon all cell functions.

5. By means of antibodies (globulins) and the white cells, blood forms an important defence system against disease.

6. By means of platelets and fibrin clot-forming proteins in the blood, blood loss following injury is controlled, and initiation and maintenance of repair of damage are carried out.

7. Blood plays an important role in the regulation of normal body temperature.

3. Dental Anatomy and Physiology

Teeth are hard, highly calcified structures, supported in each jaw by a bony socket called an 'alveolus'. Each tooth consists of a crown which is the part visible in the mouth, and one or more roots in sockets in the jawbone. The crown and root(s) join at the 'neck' (cervical margin) of the tooth (see below). Each jaw normally has a complete arch of teeth, comprising four types: incisors, canines (cuspids), premolars (bi-cuspids) and molars.

Incisors are used for incising (cutting off) portions of food, and are situated at the front of each dental arch. The crowns of the incisors have a single cutting edge.

Canines have a pointed crown which is designed for gripping and shearing smaller food portions from larger pieces. They are situated next to the incisors at the front of the mouth.

Premolars and molars have broad biting surfaces, formed from raised cusps with pits and fissures between them. When the upper and lower molar and premolar teeth bite together, they form a grinding surface capable of breaking down lumps of food into smaller, soft, moistened, swallowable pieces. The anterior teeth also perform an important role in speech and development of facial appearance.

In the adult, there are thirty-two permanent teeth (Fig. 3.1b); sixteen in each jaw, eight on each side of the jaw: two incisors, one canine, two premolars and three molars. Children have primary (deciduous or 'milk) teeth, which are replaced by the permanent dentition as growth progresses. The deciduous dentition consists of twenty teeth, ten in each jaw, five on each side. They are grouped as follows: two incisors, one canine and two molars in each half of each jaw (Fig. 3.1a). The change from deciduous to permanent dentition begins at around six years of age (see Chapter 7 on 'Children and Dentistry').

STRUCTURE OF TEETH

The main component of a tooth is a bone-like material called 'dentine'. Over the crown dentine there is a layer of a hard, calcified tissue called 'enamel' which, because of its hardness, is well suited to chewing.

Roots of teeth are covered by a thin layer of substance termed 'cementum'. This bone-like material is especially adapted to anchor the tooth into its bony socket. The enamel and cementum meet at the cervical margin or neck of the tooth at a boundary called the cemento-enamel (or amelo-cemental) junction (amelo=enamel). The dentine encloses the nerves and blood vessels responsible for a tooth's vitality. This tissue is called the 'dental pulp', and it

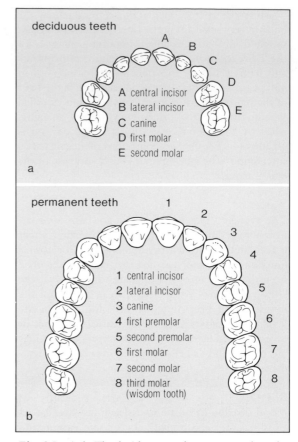

Fig. 3.1a & b *The deciduous and permanent dental arches; grouping of deciduous and permanent teeth.*

is contained within the pulp chamber of the crown and the pulp canal of the root. These two chambers are continuous. The blood vessels and nerves enter into the pulp chamber through a small foramen in the root apex, called the 'apical foramen' (see Fig. 3.2).

Enamel

Enamel is the most highly mineralised tissue in the body, hence it is very resistant to destruction. Teeth may be the only recognisable feature of a human body after a disaster (such as fire), so that identification of individuals may rely upon characteristics recorded from their surviving teeth.

Enamel does not contain nerves or blood vessels and is therefore totally insensitive to pain. Furthermore, unlike most other tissues in the body, it cannot undergo repair. Thus, enamel loss caused by dental decay or other injury is permanent. Microscopically,

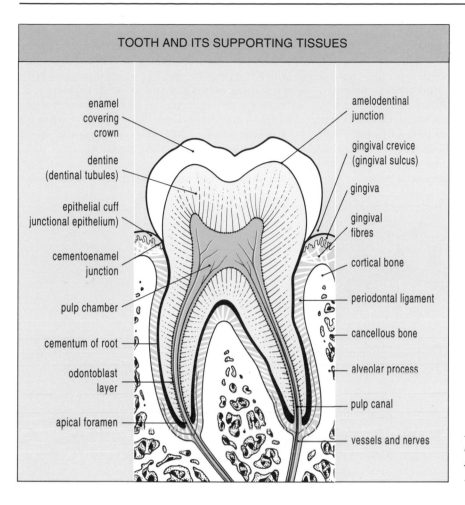

TOOTH AND ITS SUPPORTING TISSUES

enamel covering crown

dentine (dentinal tubules)

epithelial cuff junctional epithelium)

cementoenamel junction

pulp chamber

cementum of root

odontoblast layer

apical foramen

amelodentinal junction

gingival crevice (gingival sulcus)

gingiva

gingival fibres

cortical bone

periodontal ligament

cancellous bone

alveolar process

pulp canal

vessels and nerves

Fig. 3.2 Cross-section of a molar, showing its structure. See also Fig. 9.1.

enamel is composed of solid rods of mineral, called 'prisms', which intertwine with each other for strength. Prisms are held together by an interprismatic cement.

Dentine

Dentine (ivory) is a bone-like porous material, but much softer than enamel. It contains the processes of living cells which originate in the dental pulp, called 'odontoblasts', and occupy dentinal tubules which give dentine its porous nature. The odontoblasts maintain the vitality and health of dentine, and make it a highly sensitive tissue. Any stimulus, for example temperature, touch or sweet substances, produces only a sensation of pain. Normally, the sensitive dentine is protected from such painful stimuli by the resistant insensitive enamel, Dentine, by nature of its structure, has a slightly elastic, shock-

absorbing quality, which supports the enamel and resists a tooth being shattered during use.

Pulp

Pulp consists of cells, nerves and blood vessels. The combination of these provides nourishment and sensitivity to teeth. The blood vessels and nerves pass through the apical foramen of the root apex, and communicate with the vessels and nerves of that jaw. The dentinal surface of the pulp is covered by odontoblasts which transmit long processes into the tubules of dentine. The odontoblasts originally produce the dentine and retain the ability to do so. Therefore when an area of dentine becomes affected by dental decay or irritant filling materials, the odontoblasts generate a secondary, reparative layer of dentine at the pulpal surface. Secondary dentine is normally produced very slowly throughout life.

35

Hence in older people root canals and pulp chambers are smaller than those of the young.

Supporting tissues of the teeth

A tooth is supported in a bony socket (alveolus), which is an extension of the basic bone of the jaw. Alveolar bone is only present where a tooth is present. It disappears (resorbs) gradually after tooth removal, leading eventually to 'gum shrinkage' as seen most obviously in patients who have been without any teeth (edentulous) for several years.

An alveolus consists of a layer of dense, cortical bone which lines the socket inside and outside, enclosing a layer of spongy or 'cancellous' bone which is richly vascular. The calcium salts of bone are constantly removed and replaced, enabling it to be strong and rigid, yet not so brittle as to fracture easily. This remodelling helps bone to adapt to changing forces, and makes orthodontic tooth movement possible (see also Chapter 8).

The root surface of a tooth is covered with cementum. Between the cortical bone of the socket

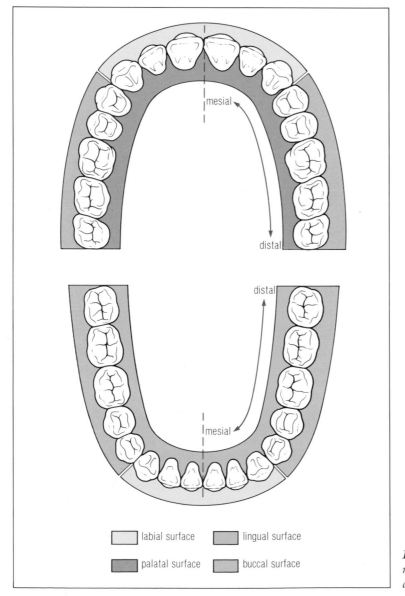

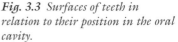

labial surface   lingual surface

palatal surface   buccal surface

Fig. 3.3 *Surfaces of teeth in relation to their position in the oral cavity.*

wall and the cementum of the tooth root run slightly coiled fibres of a non-elastic material called 'collagen'. These fibres are attached to the alveolar bone on one side, and into the cementum of the root on the other. The tooth is thus anchored into the socket.

The collagen fibres form the 'periodontal ligament'. Their arrangement is organised such that vertical pressures on the teeth are resisted. A fluid between the collagen fibres acts as a shock-absorbing cushion to the movement of a tooth in its socket, made possible by slight uncoiling of the collagen fibres. This mechanisms ensures that a tooth does not shatter in normal use.

The outer surface of the alveolar bone is covered with an attached gum (gingiva). This gingival tissue becomes continuous with the flexible mucous membrane lining the oral cavity of the buccal sulcus (or 'vestibule'). Around each tooth the gingiva forms a 'cuff' which grips the cervical margin of the tooth at the cemento-enamel junctions. This 'cuff' is held in place by a gingival group of periodontal ligament fibres, and prevents food from passing into the periodontal ligament. The bulbous nature of the tooth itself directs food away from this delicate gingival margin. The potential space between tooth and gingival margin is called the 'gingival crevice' or 'gingival sulcus'. Fluid from the periodontal ligament flows through this space helping to cleanse the area and prevent periodontal disease. Figure 3.2 depicts the structure and supporting tissues of a tooth (a molar is taken as an example).

ANATOMY OF TEETH

Teeth have a number of surfaces (Fig. 3.3). The outer surfaces of the molars and premolars face the buccinator muscle, hence this is known as the *buccal surface*. The outer surface of the incisors and canines faces the lip, and it is therefore called *labial*. The inner surface of the upper teeth is adjacent to the palate (*palatal*), and the tongue lies on the inner side of the lower teeth (*lingual*). The tooth surface which faces towards the midline is known as *mesial*, and that facing towards the back of the dental arch is known as *distal*. The flat, biting surface of molars and premolars is called the *occlusal surface*, and the cutting edge of incisors and canines is called the *incisal edge*. Where two adjacent teeth touch in the dental arch, they form a *contact point*.

Permanent teeth

Permanent incisors have a single root and a spade-shaped crown. The upper are wider than the lower. Permanent canines have large, bulbous, roughly conical crowns, and one stout, long root. Maxillary are larger than mandibular canines. The maxillary first premolar usually has two roots: one buccal and one palatal. All other premolars usually have a single root. Premolars are sometimes called 'bicuspids' because they have two cusps. In the maxilla, premolars have buccal and palatal cusps of a roughly equal size, whilst in the mandible the lingual cusp is much smaller than the buccal cusp.

Maxillary molars have three roots: two buccal and one palatal. Mandibular molars have two roots: one mesial and one distal. Maxillary molar crowns have four cusps: two buccal and two palatal. The overall crown shape, when viewed from the occlusal surface, is slightly lozenge-shaped , and a prominent oblique ridge crosses the occlusal surface between the mesiopalatal and distobuccal cusps. Between cusps there are fissures and pits. The maxillary first permanent molar has an additional cusp as an extension to the mesiopalatal cusp, called 'Carabelli's tubercle'. Mandibular molars have two roots, one mesial and one distal. The crowns when viewed from their occlusal surface, are roughly square or oblong in shape. Mandibular first permanent molars are the largest of all molar teeth and have five cusps: three buccal and two lingual. Mandibular second and third molars have four cusps: two buccal and two lingual (permanent teeth; Fig. 3.4).

Deciduous teeth

Apart from premolars, which are not present in the deciduous dentition, the crowns and roots of deciduous teeth roughly resemble their permanent counterparts but with some differences (Fig. 3.4) (see also Chapter 7).

Development of teeth

As early on as forty-two days after conception, the first signs of tooth development may be seen in the human embryo. In the region of the primitive oral cavity specialised cells line up and form into an arch called the 'dental lamina' (lamina = sheet) which corresponds to the future dental arch of each jaw. From this lamina, 'buds' of cells develop on the palatal and lingual sides, one for each deciduous tooth, and shortly afterwards a bud for each permanent tooth develops. The buds form an enamel organ, and the innermost layer of its cells develops into ameloblasts which eventually produce enamel. Once the ameloblasts have formed, they induce the adjacent connective tissue cells to form a dental papilla, which in turn produces dentine and tooth pulp. The enamel organ and dental papilla are

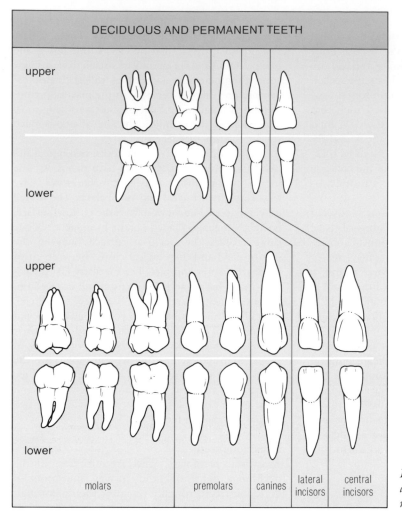

DECIDUOUS AND PERMANENT TEETH

upper

lower

upper

lower

molars   premolars   canines   lateral incisors   central incisors

Fig. 3.4 *Shapes of deciduos teeth and permanent teeth and their roots.*

enclosed in a fibrous sack called a 'follicle'.

Ultimately, each formed tooth pushes through the gum into the oral cavity (eruption). The mechanism whereby teeth move and erupt into the mouth is not understood, but factors such as root growth, alveolar bond growth and the blood pressure inside the developing pulp are thought to play a part. Most permanent teeth erupt before their roots are fully formed, the apical area of the root still being open. Root completion occurs approximately three years after tooth eruption. Permanent third molars and canines, however, usually have completed roots when they erupt. Deciduous teeth start to erupt at approximately six months of age, and all have erupted by the age of two years. There is further discussion on deciduous teeth and tooth development in Chapter 7.

Occlusion and articulation of teeth

The upper and lower teeth are said to be occluding when they close together. Articulation is the movement of the upper teeth against the lower. Occlusion is a stationary contact, whereas articulation is a moving contact. Normally, the upper teeth form a slightly larger dental arch than the lower. Therefore, in normal occlusion the upper anterior teeth are slightly in front of the lower. Similarly, the upper posterior teeth occlude with their buccal surface slightly outside the buccal surface of the lower teeth (Fig. 3.5a).

The centre line between the upper central incisors and that between the lower should coincide when the teeth are in normal occlusion. As the maxillary incisors are wider than the mandibular, each tooth occludes with two teeth in the opposite jaw

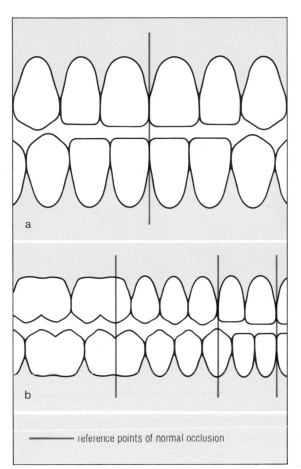

——— reference points of normal occlusion

Fig. 3.5 a & b Occlusion and articulation of teeth; upper and lower incisors and canines; upper and lower premolars and molars.

(see Fig. 3.5b). Also, the mandibular canine occludes in front of the maxillary, and the mesio-buccal cusps of the maxillary first permanent molar occludes in the buccal groove between the two buccal cusps of the mandibular first permanent molar (Fig. 3.5b). Chapter 8 discusses in detail types of occlusion and articulation.

Dental record charts are discussed on page 14.

THE SKULL

The skull is divided into two main parts: the part enclosing the brain is called the 'neurocranium', and the remainder forms the face.

Eight bones collectively form the neurocranium. These are the frontal, occipital, sphenoid, ethmoid, the two parietal and the two temporal bones. The neurocranium is perfectly adapted for protecting the delicate tissues of the brain. The sides are sloped, minimising the impact of a blow to the area. There are no sharp corners or angles, and each bone fits the neighbouring bone like a jigsaw puzzle piece, forming a rigid entity. These interlocking joints are called 'sutures'. The floor of the neurocranium is formed by the occipital, sphenoid and ethmoid bones. The lateral aspects are formed by the paired temporal and parietal bones (roughly square-shaped and slightly convex), and the front of the neurocranium is composed of the large unpaired frontal bone; this forms the forehead and contains airspaces called 'frontal sinuses' (Fig. 3.6 a, b, c).

The occipital bone articulates with the first cervical vertebra by two small and rounded 'condyles'. It is easily identified by the large opening called 'foramen magnum', through which the spinal cord travels to join the brain (Fig. 3.7).

39

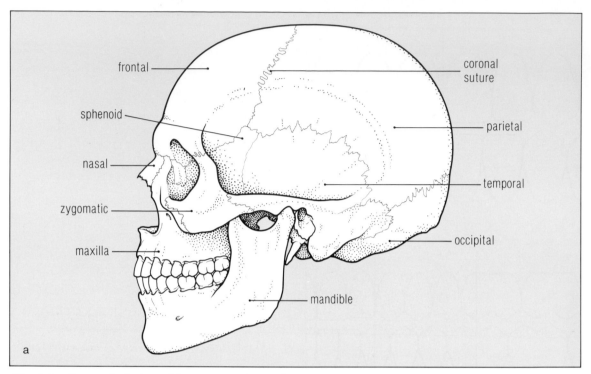

Fig. 3.6 a *Bone articulations of the neurocranium: side view.*

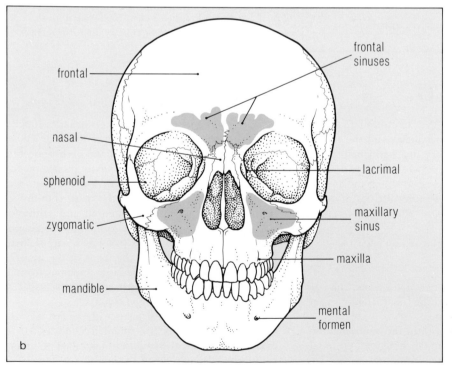

Fig. 3.6 b *Bone articulations of the neurocranium: front view.*

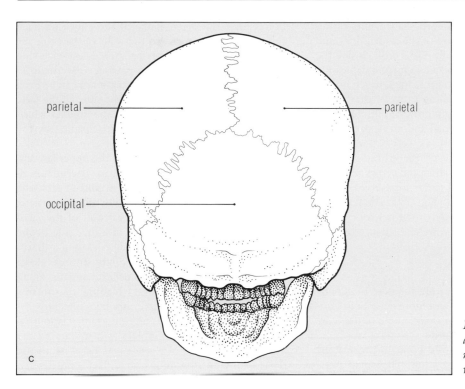

Fig. 3.6 c *Bone articulations of the neurocranium: back view.*

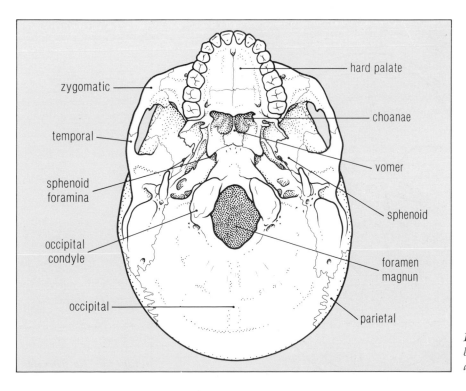

Fig. 3.7 *The occipital bone of the skull and its articulations.*

The sphenoid bone is bird-shaped and rather complex, forming the centre of the cranial floor and also contributing to the walls of the orbit. Inside the skull, the sphenoid bone contains a marked depression called the 'sella turcica' (turkish saddle), which houses the pituitary gland controlling many of the body's chemical processes, including growth (Fig. 3.8).

The ethmoid bone is small and forms part of the floor of the neurocranium, as well as part of the nose. The unique feature of the ethmoid is the cribriform plate, through which the nerves responsible for the sense of smell (olfactory nerves) travel from the nose to the brain (Fig. 3.9). The temporal bones form part of the side of the neurocranium, and house the delicate hearing and balance sensory apparatus.

The face

The remaining skull bones form the face. In general they are rather specialised and more delicate in construction, varying greatly in shape. Some of them are important for the DSA to know.

The vomer is an unpaired bone and forms the lower part of the nasal septum. The small nasal bones form the bridge of the nose. The lacrimal bones are found in the medial aspects of the orbit and are the smallest bones of the face. The zygomatic bones form the prominence of the cheek on each side, contributing partly to the walls of the orbit. By an extension which passes backwards on each side they join a similar extension passing forwards from the temporal bone, to form a zygomatic arch. Each arch gives shape and support to the sides of the face, as well as attachment for some of the muscles which operate the jaw. The hard palate is formed by the palatine bones and maxilla.

The maxilla on each side forms the upper jaw and is a fixed part of the facial skeleton. It contains all upper teeth in their sockets. The maxilla of each side is joined together below the nose by the hard palate, and also forms part of the lateral wall of the nasal cavity and floor of the orbit. On either side of the nasal cavity the maxilla is hollow, enclosing a maxillary sinus or antrum. The maxillary sinuses, along with the frontal sinuses, have a delicate mucosal lining which may become inflamed leading to sinusitis when there is an upper respiratory tract infection.

The maxillary sinus has an important relationship to the roots of the premolars and molars of the maxilla. The apices of these roots lie close to the floor of the antrum. Thus, maxillary sinusitis can lead to the feeling of toothache in the adjacent teeth. Furthermore, during tooth removal the maxillary antrum floor may be perforated, creating an

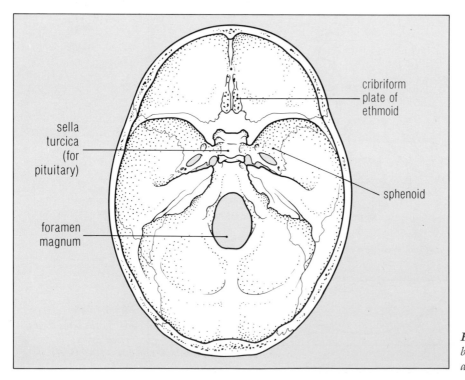

sella turcica (for pituitary)

foramen magnum

cribriform plate of ethmoid

sphenoid

Fig. 3.8 *The sphenoid bone of the skull and its articulations.*

opening between the maxillary sinus and the mouth. This 'oro-antral fistula' must be closed surgically.

The mandible is the single bone of the lower jaw, capable of moving so that the mouth opens and closes (Fig. 3.10). It articulates on each side with the glenoid fossa of the temporal bone, and has a roughly horseshoe-shaped horizontal body as well as two vertical portions at each side (rami) which project

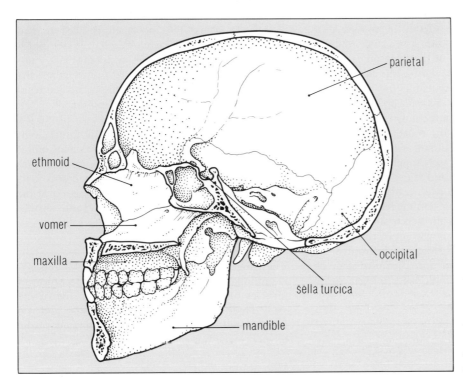

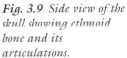

Fig. 3.9 *Side view of the skull showing ethmoid bone and its articulations.*

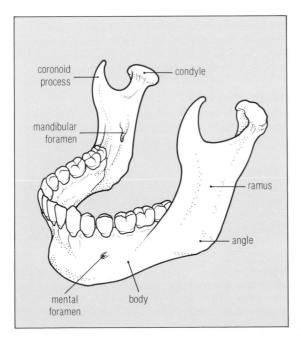

Fig. 3.10 *The mandible, the single bone of the lower jaw.(see also Fig. 3.21a).*

43

upwards. At the top of each ramus there are two projections: the condyle, which forms the temporo-mandibular joint at its articulation with the temporal bone, and the coronoid process which is in front of the condyle and serves as a muscle attachment. The junction between the body and each ramus occurs at the angle of the mandible. On the inner surface of each ramus there is a hole leading to a canal running through the entire length of the body on each side of the mandible. This is known as the mandibular foramen and canal, and transmits the nerves and vessels responsible for blood supply and innervation to and from the mandibular teeth. On the outer surface of the body between the roots of the two permanent premolars there is the mental foramen transmitting the nerves and vessels supplying the lower lip on that side with blood and sensation.

The temporomandibular joint, formed between the condyle of the mandible and the temporal bone, lies at the base of the skull. When the mouth is closed, the condyle head moves out of the glenoid fossa and rests on a bony projection in front of it, known as the articular eminence. The initial stage of opening the mouth is a simple hinge movement of the tempormandibular joint, rotating around an axis which passes between the two mandibular condyle heads on each side (Fig. 3.11).

To open the mouth wider than this simple hinge movement permits, each condyle head must move forwards, out of the glenoid fossa and onto the articular eminence. This movement is called 'translatory'. Thus, unlike many joints, the temporo-mandibular joint can undergo both hinge and translatory movements. Jaw closure occurs when the condyle returns to the glenoid fossa, and the teeth are brought together by the hinge movement.

During mastication, side movements of the jaw are permitted by one temporomandibular joint undergoing hinge and translatory movements out of the glenoid fossa, while the opposite joint remains within the glenoid fossa. When the jaw returns to its original central position, the shearing action of the posterior teeth shreds a bolus of food into smaller particles.

MUSCLES OF MASTICATION

The movements of the mandible and temporo-mandibular joints are controlled by the powerful muscles of mastication, four on each side of the skull. Three are responsible for jaw closure, and one for the opening and translatory movements of the temporomandibular joints.

Lateral pterygoid

This muscle originates behind the maxilla and inserts into the front of the condyle of the mandible. When both muscles work together, they pull the mandible forwards by a translatory movement of the condyle onto the articular eminence (Fig. 3.12). If one muscle acts alone, it swings the jaw to the opposite side.

Medial pterygoid

This muscle also arises from behind the maxilla, and inserts into the inner surface of the ramus and angle of the mandible. Its action is to close jaw (Fig. 3.12).

Masseter

This muscle originates from the zygomatic arch and inserts into the outside of the ramus and angle of the mandible. When it contracts, it closes the jaw (Fig. 3.13).

Temporalis

The temporalis muscle arises from the side of the skull and inserts into the coronoid process of the mandible. When it contracts, it pulls the jaw backwards and the teeth are brought together (Fig. 3.14).

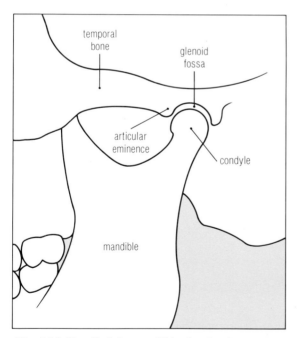

Fig. 3.11 *Detail of the mandible, showing bone articulations that perform the hinge movement of the tempomandibular joint.*

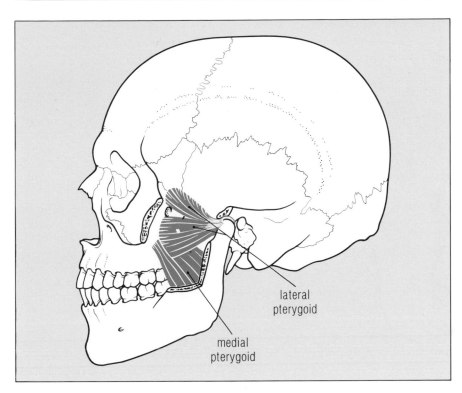

Fig. 3.12 Muscles of mastication: medial and lateral pterygoids.

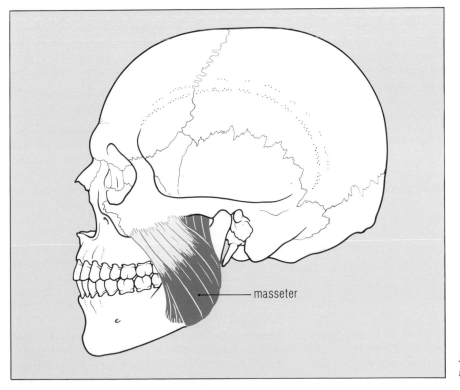

Fig. 3.13 Muscles of mastication: masseter.

45

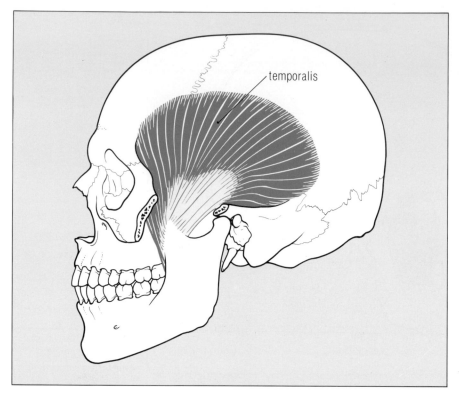

Fig. 3.14 Muscles of mastication: temporalis.

THE ORAL CAVITY

The oral cavity is divided into two regions. The region between the lips or cheeks and the teeth is called the 'outer vestibule' or 'buccal sulcus'. The cheeks and lips are attached to the jaw by strands of fibrous tissue, each called a 'frenum'. The space between the inner surfaces of the teeth on each side is known as the 'inner vestibule' or 'oral cavity proper' (Fig. 3.15).

The lining of the cheeks, roof of the mouth (palate), floor of the mouth and tongue, is formed by a layer of epithelium moistened by saliva. This is the oral mucous membrane, richly supplied with blood which gives it its pink/red colour. It is also richly supplied with nerves, hence its extreme sensitivity. The moisture is derived from the salivary glands.

Salivary glands

These are of two types: major and minor (Fig. 3.16). The minor glands lie inside the mouth, scattered throughout the mucous membrane lining the oral cavity, secreting saliva directly onto the mucosal surface. The major glands are situated outside the mouth, and their secretions are conveyed into the mouth by ducts which open through the oral mucosa. The major glands are paired on each side of the head. There are three pairs:

Parotid

Each of these is situated behind and over the outer surface of the ramus of the mandible. The parotid duct passes forwards from the gland, runs onto the surface of the masseter muscle in the cheek, and turns towards the mouth where it opens through the mucosa opposite the second maxillary molar.

Submandibular

These are situated on each side of the inner surface of the angle of the mandible. The submandibular duct runs forwards and opens into the floor of the mouth, behind the lower incisor teeth.

Sublingual

These also lie under the floor of the mouth, anterior to the submandibular gland, beneath the tongue. There are several small ducts from each of these glands, opening directly into the floor of the mouth.

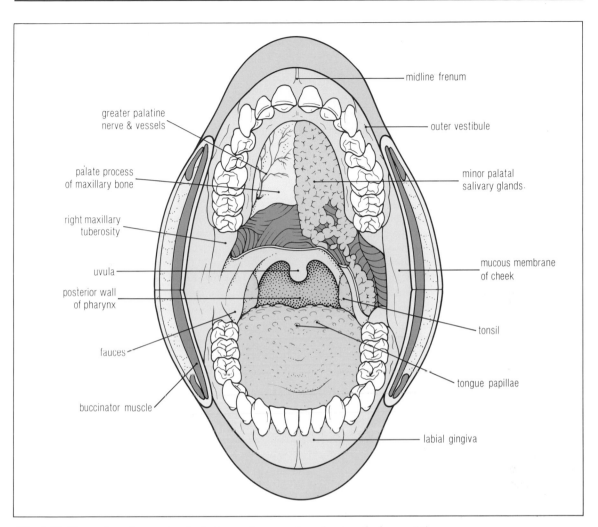

Fig. 3.15 *The oral cavity: anatomical view and cross sections showing the layers of the mucosa.*

The minor glands (see Fig. 3.16) are generally responsible for maintaining moisture of the mucous membrane, whereas the major glands product large amounts of saliva in response to food intake. The flow is controlled automatically by the autonomic nervous system. Saliva has two main functions:

Protection
By its chemical composition, saliva is a lubricating agent which maintains the health of the oral mucous membrane and teeth. Many harmful bacteria are destroyed by an antibody contained in the saliva. Also, teeth are partly protected from decay and acid attack by agents in saliva which neutralise and dilute the acidic concentration.

Patients suffering from dry mouth and deficiency of saliva (following certain drug treatments, or as a complication of rheumatoid arthritis), find speaking, eating and swallowing dry food, very difficult. The oral mucosa becomes susceptible to infections, and teeth decay rapidly.

Digestion
Saliva contains the enzyme amylase (ptyalin) which initiates digestion of carbohydrates. This is completed when food reaches the duodenum and small intestine.

47

The roof of the mouth

The roof of the mouth is formed by the hard and soft palates. The hard palate is formed by the palatine process of the maxilla and the palatine bones on each side (see Fig. 3.15). Behind the hard palate lies the soft palate composed of movable soft tissue. It seals the back of the nose from the oral cavity during swallowing, preventing food from entering the nasal cavity.

The tongue

The tongue has important functions involving taste, speech and swallowing. It also acts with the cheeks in maintaining the position of food between the upper and lower teeth during chewing, and has a cleansing action by removing particles of food from the teeth or buccal sulcus after swallowing. The root of the tongue is associated with the muscles forming the floor of the oral cavity. Its anterior, highly mobile part is connected to the floor of the mouth by a fibrous band, the lingual frenum. The mucous membrane covering the upper surface of the tongue is a highly specialised, thickened mucosa, covered in papillae which give the surface a coarse texture. These facilitate its ability to manipulate food and clean the surfaces of the teeth. The undersurface of the tongue is covered by a thin, delicate mucous membrane, rich in blood vessels, which enables some drugs in a sublingual tablet form to be rapidly absorbed into the blood stream. The best example is the glyceryl trinitrate tablet for relief of cardiac pain (angina). Some of the surface papillae are specialised for taste perception. The four basic tastes distinguished are bitter, sweet, salt and sour. Taste sensation, coupled with smell, gives the combined effect of flavour.

MUSCLES OF FACIAL EXPRESSION

This sheet-like layer of muscle surrounds the eyes, nose, mouth and ears, and forms the cheeks, fore-

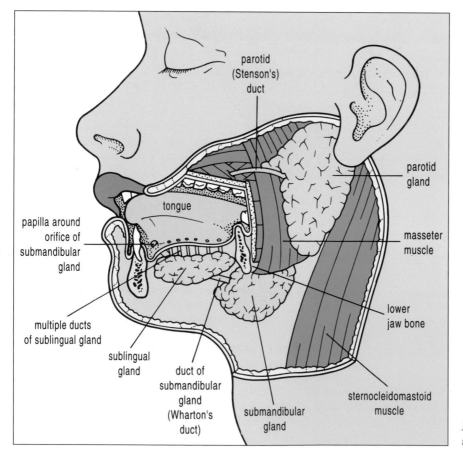

Fig. 3.16 Major and minor salivary glands.

head, scalp and neck. The component parts have an origin attached to bone, and they are inserted into the facial skin. Thus, contraction of the muscle moves the skin. The muscles work as constrictors and dilators of an opening. Around the eyes lies the orbicularis oculi, and around the mouth the orbicularis oris (Fig. 3.17). Thin muscle bands extend from the zygomatic bone to the cheek skin (zygomaticus muscles). The muscle of the cheeks is the buccinator (buccina = trumpet). This is attached to the alveolar processes of the maxilla and mandible above and below, and thereby forms a limit to the buccal sulcus on each side. Its fibres, with the orbicularis oris, form the muscles of the lips. It is also continuous with the muscular wall of the pharynx behind. The buccinator plays an important role with the tongue in maintaining a bolus of food between the working teeth during mastication, and in directing the bolus towards the back of the mouth prior to swallowing.

NERVES OF THE HEAD AND NECK

The nervous system is divided into two parts: central (the brain and spinal cord) and peripheral (the nerves that travel to serve all parts of the body). Information travels into and out of the central nervous system along these nerve pathways. Sensations reaching the brain in sensory nerves convey information regarding touch, temperature and pain. Information leaving the brain in motor nerves operates muscles or glands. The brain has twelve pairs of cranial nerves which convey sensory and motor information. Those specifically affecting the dental regions of the head and neck are the fifth, seventh, ninth and twelfth cranial nerves.

Trigeminal (fifth)

This is a most important nerve, as it conveys sensory information from the oral cavity, including teeth, gums, tongue, lips and cheeks. It also conveys the motor supply for the muscles of mastication.

Facial (seventh)

This is the motor nerve for the muscle of facial expression, and the motor supply which controls the secretions of the submandibular and sublingual salivary glands. It also conveys the sense of taste from the anterior two-thirds of the tongue.

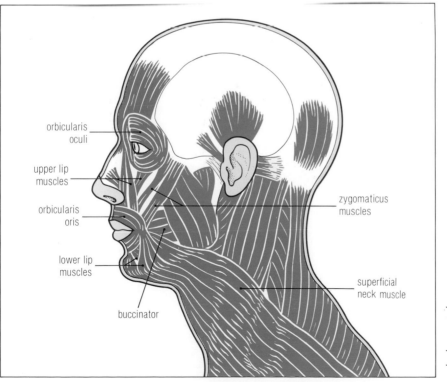

orbicularis
oculi

upper lip
muscles

orbicularis
oris

lower lip
muscles

buccinator

zygomaticus
muscles

superficial
neck muscle

Fig. 3.17 Muscles of facial expression, surrounding the eyes, nose, mouth and ears, forming the cheeks, forehead, scalp and neck.

Glossopharyngeal (ninth)

This nerve conveys the motor information to the parotid salivary glands, and sensory information from the pharynx. The sense of taste from the posterior one-third of the tongue is carried to the brain via this nerve.

Hypoglossal (twelfth)

This nerve conveys the motor function to the muscle within the tongue.

Sensation from the oral cavity

The oral cavity (teeth and jaws, their associated mucous membrane and skin) is supplied with sensory nerves from the trigeminal cranial nerve on each side. Taste is the only sensation not conveyed by the trigeminal nerve, being conveyed instead by the facial and glossopharyngeal nerves to the brain. The trigeminal nerve consists of three divisions (Fig. 3.18):

1. *Ophthalmic*, supplying structures associated with the eyes.

2. *Maxillary*, serving the upper jaw and teeth, as well as the upper part of the facial skin. It conveys touch, temperature and pain from these regions to the brain. This division has no motor function.

3. *Mandibular*, with a motor and sensory function. The motor nerve fibres supply the muscles of mastication. The sensory nerve fibres convey information to the brain from the lower jaw and teeth, as well as from the associated mucous membrane and skin of the lower part of the face.

NERVE SUPPLY TO TEETH AND SUPPORTING STRUCTURES

Operative procedures on teeth, such as removing decay or tooth extraction, are extremely painful if performed without anaesthesia. Usually, patients receive injection of anaesthetic which temporarily stops sensory nerves conducting impulses to the brain. Knowledge of the nerves and their position for each tooth is necessary, so that pain may be blocked during an operation. This is achieved by

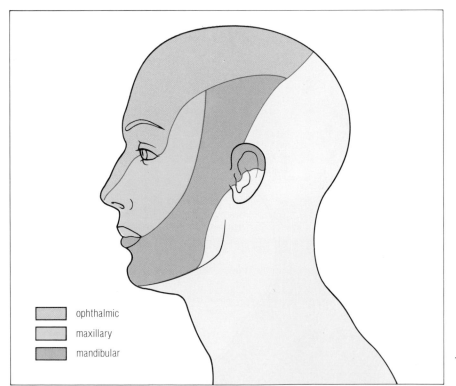

ophthalmic

maxillary

mandibular

Fig. 3.18 Sensation from the oral cavity: the trigeminal nerve and its three division.

accurate deposition of local anaesthetic solution (see also Chapter 11 and 12).

Sensory information from dental structures is conveyed by three different nerve networks. A network of nerves is called a 'plexus'. Fine nerve fibres collect into enlarging bundles from each plexus and form the major nerve pathways. The inner plexus serves the lingual or palatal bone and gingivae. The outer plexus serves the buccal or labial bone and gingivae, and the dental plexus serves the tooth pulp, dentine and periodontal ligament (Fig. 3.19).

Maxilla

In the upper jaw, the dental plexus forms the anterior, middle and posterior dental nerves. These nerves run within the maxillary bone and eventually join the maxillary division of the trigeminal nerve, and thence to the brain. The outer plexus of the incisors and canines forms the infraorbital nerve, which also supplies the skin of the face and upper lips of this region. The intraorbital nerve joins the maxillary nerve by entering the infraorbital foramen (Fig. 3.20a). In the region of the premolars and molars of the maxilla, the outer plexus forms the buccal nerves which also supply the skin and the cheeks of this region. The buccal nerves reach the brain by joining the mandibular nerve.

Anteriorly, the inner plexus forms the long sphenopalatine nerve which joins the maxillary nerve by passing upwards into the incisive foramen and canal. Posteriorly, the inner plexus forms the greater palatine nerve which also joins the large maxillary nerve, through the greater palatine foramen, at the back of the maxilla (Fig. 3.20b & c).

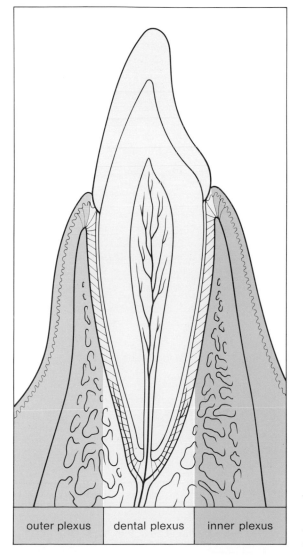

| outer plexus | dental plexus | inner plexus |

Fig. 3.19 *The three nerve networks (plexuses) that convey sensory information from the dental structures.*

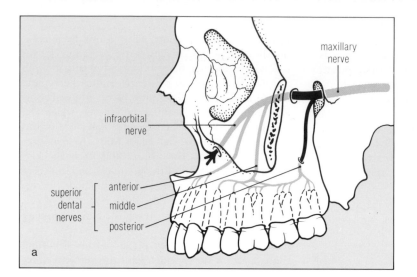

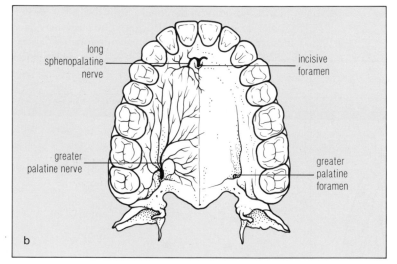

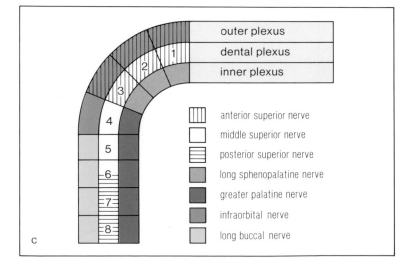

Fig. 3.20 a ,b ,c Nerve supply to the maxilla.

Mandible

In the lower jaw, the dental plexus of all teeth on each side forms the inferior dental nerve, which runs inside the mandibular body beneath the teeth roots and continues inside the ramus, until it reaches the mandibular foramen where it joins the mandibular division of the trigeminal nerve. The labial plexus, associated with the incisors, canine and premolars on each side (including the skin of the lower lip), forms the mental nerve which joins the inferior dental nerve by passing though the mental foramen of the mandible (Fig. 3.21a).

The buccal plexus, associated with the mandibular molars, forms the buccal nerves which join the mandibular nerve with the inferior dental nerve.

The lingual plexus forms the lingual nerve on each side, which also joins the mandibular nerve. Thus, all sensations from the mandibular dental structures reach the brain via the mandibular nerve, by travelling in the lingual, inferior dental, or long buccal nerves (Fig. 3.21b).

BLOOD SUPPLY TO THE HEAD AND NECK

The head and neck, including the face, teeth and jaws, are supplied by branches of the external carotid artery. Veins draining these parts eventually join the superior vena cava (see Fig. 2.4). The arteries and veins to each component run along with the nerves, and usually have the same name.

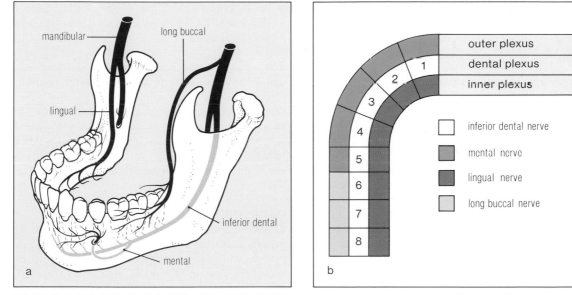

Fig. 3.21 a & b Nerve supply to the mandible.

4. The Medical History

Every patient treated in a dental surgery should have a medical history taken. Oral diseases may be influenced by systemic disorders. The medical history will also determine the type of dental treatment and anaesthesia needed, the use of drugs, and any prophylactic precautions required against cross-infection (*Fig. 4.1*). The dentist may obtain the medical history by allowing patients to talk about their medical problems, guiding them with questions that will lead to a relevant history. Information must be sought concerning:

A - Anaemia
B - Bleeding tendency
C - Cardiorespiratory disease (heart and lung problems)
D - Drug use and allergies
E - Endocrine diseases, especially diabetes
F - Fits or faints
G - Gastrointestinal disease
H - History of previous operations or admissions to hospital
I - Infections and infectious diseases
J - Jaundice and liver disease
K - Kidney disease
L - Likelihood of pregnancy

ANAEMIA

Anaemia may be a contraindication to general anaesthesia, as the ability of blood to carry oxygen to the brain and other tissues is reduced. Sickle cell anaemia is of particular importance and tends to be commonest among black patients. General anaesthesia should never be given to patients with sickle cell anaemia unless in hospital, as it may induce a dangerous crisis. Other types of anaemia may predispose to mouth ulcers, a sore tongue, angular cheilitis and thrush.

BLEEDING TENDENCY

Surgery can be dangerous in patients with a bleeding tendency. Local anaesthetic injections may also be dangerous. They can cause tissue bleeding extensive enough to cause swelling around the throat, which may choke the patient.

Some drugs may worsen the bleeding tendency and are, therefore, contraindicated. Aspirin, for example, should not be used in such patients.

The normal mechanisms that stop bleeding involve the blood vessels which automatically contract slightly, the blood platelets which, to a certain extent, block the site of damage and release coagulation factors, and coagulation factors themselves. Coagulation factors are plasma proteins in an inactive state until there is tissue damage. With tissue damage a chain reaction occurs, in which the factors are activated and eventually causes fibrinogen to change to fibrin that forms a blood clot (*Fig. 4.2*). Patients can have a bleeding tendency if any one of these mechanisms is faulty. Bleeding is mostly caused by:

- A defect of platelets (thrombocytopenia), such as occurs in leukaemia.
- Interference with blood coagulation by anticoagulants (warfarin). These patients may carry a warning card.
- Defective production of clotting factors due to liver disease.
- An inherited lack of one of the clotting factors (haemophilia). These patients should be carrying a warning card.

The management of patients with a bleeding tendency involves avoiding injury wherever possible (care should be taken when handling scalpels, forceps and needles), and replacing the missing platelet or clotting factor before surgery. Thus, if oral surgery is required in a leukaemic patient a platelet transfusion is given, while in a haemophilic patient the missing coagulant is administered (usually factor VIII).

CARDIORESPIRATORY DISEASE

Cardiac disease may well be a contraindication to general anaesthesia. This is particularly the case in patients who are suffering from severe angina, or in those with a recent history of a heart attack (myocardial infarction or coronary thrombosis).

Patients suffering from diseases of the heart valves, especially those with mitral valve stenosis following rheumatic fever and those with a congenital heart disease, are at risk of developing infective endocarditis after dental treatment. In endocarditis, bacteria from the mouth (such as *Streptococcus viridans*) may enter the blood stream during tooth extraction, scaling, or other procedures where there is gingival bleeding, and settle onto the defective area causing serious infection (*Fig. 4.3*). Antibiotic prophylaxis must, therefore, be given before dental treatment commences (page 108). Respiratory disease, such as chronic bronchitis, may be another contraindication to general anaesthesia.

DISORDER	CONSIDERATIONS
Anaemia	Care with general anaesthesia.
Bleeding tendency	Care with surgery, infections, aspirin.
Cardiorespiratory disease	Antibiotic cover to prevent infective endocarditis. Care with general anaesthesia.
Drug use or allergies	Drug interactions or allergies
Endocrine disease (diabetes)	Keep blood sugar level up. Do not interfere with meals.
Fits and faints	Be prepared to deal with them.
Gastrointestinal disease	Care of vomiting with general anaesthesia.
History of previous operations	Frequently repeated halothane general anaesthesia should be avoided.
Infections	Precautions against cross-infection.
Jaundice or liver disease	Care with drugs, bleeding tendency, risk of infection.
Kidney disease	Care with drugs and bleeding tendency.
Likelihood of pregnancy	Care with drugs (including general anaesthesia) and X-rays.

Fig. 4.1 Main reasons for taking a patient's medical history.

damage to blood vessel

↓

blood vessel contracts and blood flow slows down

↓

clotting factors activated

↓

platelets stick to area of damage

↓

prothrombin activated

↓

thrombin

↓

fibrinogen

converts to

↓

fibrin clot

Fig. 4.2 Mechanisms that stop bleeding.

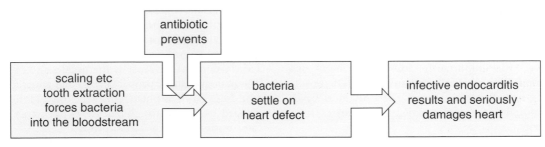

Fig. 4.3 Infective (subacute bacterial) endocarditis resulting from tooth extraction.

DRUG USE AND ALLERGIES

Certain drugs may produce oral diseases (*Fig. 4.4*), and some present serious problems in dental treatment. This is true especially of anticoagulants and corticosteroids. Patients on corticosteroids must be given steroid cover before any surgery, in order to prevent collapse. Aspirin may cause a bleeding tendency.

DRUGS	AFFECT	RESULT	MANAGEMENT
Tetracyclines	Teeth in fetus or children up to age of 8 years	Yellow, brown or grey discoloration	Use of veneers (e.g. Mastique) or crowns
Chlorhexidine mouthwash	Teeth and tooth coloured fillings	Staining	Polishing
Antidepressants	Salivary glands	Dry mouth	Salivary substitute reduce drug
Phenytoin/Cyclosporin	Gingiva	Hyperplasia	Change drug and/or perform gingivectomy
Aspirin	Mucosa if aspirin is held in mouth for a long time	Burn	Simple mouthwashes (e.g. chlorhexidine)

Fig. 4.4 *List of drugs that may produce side-effects in the mouth.*

Other drugs may interact with substances used in dentistry and antihypertensive drugs may interact with general anaesthetic agents causing a severe and dangerous fall in blood pressure. Local anaesthetics, however, are fairly safe and do not significantly interact with most drugs. A drug history is very important in that it gives a guide to a more general medical history. Some patients, for instance, are being treated for schizophrenia without openly admitting it.

Drug allergies must be investigated, particularly in relation to penicillin and anaesthetic agents. Patients allergic to penicillin may react mildly in the form of a rash, but a serious reaction may lead to anaphylactic shock and death.

Drug abuse (drug addiction) is an increasing problem. Some addicts pretend to have dental pain in order to persuade the dentist to prescribe analgesics. More importantly, addicts may be at risk from infection, especially hepatitis and AIDS, or suffering from venereal disease. The DSA must never be misled into giving advice about drugs to a patient.

ENDOCRINE DISEASE

Diabetes is the most serious endocrine disease in dentistry. The danger facing diabetics is that of missing a meal because of a delay in the surgery or pain before and after treatment. If that happens, and in case of fever or infection, the diabetes may go out of control. Thus, the DSA must always bear the particular needs of diabetic patients in mind when arranging appointments for them: early morning appointments are best.

The diabetic may develop a low sugar level in the blood (hypoglycaemia) leading to collapse, coma and possibly death. This can be prevented by ensuring that meals are taken on time or, if that is impossible, that the patient receives dental treatment as an in-patient in hospital so that the blood sugar may be maintained at normal levels by balancing the diet and providing appropriate antidiabetic treatment.

FITS AND FAINTS

It is important to know whether the patient is liable to fits or faints, as they may take place in the dental surgery. It then becomes easier and less worrying to deal with the emergency (see Chapter 15, page 155). Grand mal epilepsy is the usual cause of fits. The patient is most probably receiving anticonvulsant drugs (such as phenytoin) which should not be stopped by the dentist. Incidentally, phenytoin can cause unsightly gingival hyperplasia.

GASTROINTESTINAL DISEASE

Gastrointestinal disease is not often of particular relevance to dentistry, but patients with diseases of the small intestine (such as coeliac disease or Crohn's disease) may have difficulty in absorbing food nutrients (malabsorption) and suffer from mouth ulcers,

INFECTION	MANIFESTATIONS	PRECAUTIONS
Any respiratory or common cold virus	Respiratory infections	Sterilise equipment, wear mask and gloves
Epsein–Barr virus	Glandular fever	
Herpes simplex virus	A painful whitlow of the finger may be produced in dental staff	Sterilise equipment, wear gloves, avoid injuries from sharp instruments
Hepatitis viruses	Hepatitis and other complications such as chronic liver disease or cancer	Sterilise equipment, have vaccination, wear protective clothing, avoid injuries with sharp instruments
HIV viruses	AIDS and related syndromes	
Rubella virus	German measles in child or adult but danger to fetus in pregnancy	Female staff should be immunised against rubella

Fig. 4.5 *Prevention of transmission of viral infections in the dental surgery.*

INFECTION	MANIFESTATIONS	PRECAUTIONS
Syphilis	Primary syphilis (chancre) on finger	Sterilise equipment Wear gloves
Tuberculosis	Tuberculosis	Sterilise equipment Wear mask

Fig. 4.6 *Bacterial infections that may occasionally be transmitted in the surgery.*

a sore tongue and angular cheilitis (cracks at the angles of the mouth). Also, vomiting from any cause can be dangerous in general anaesthesia.

PREVIOUS OPERATIONS OR ADMISSIONS TO HOSPITAL

If patients have previously had a successful operation without complications, it is possible that they will have little problem in future operations (unless a new illness has developed since). In particular, if there was no severe postoperative bleeding and a good recovery was made from the anaesthetic, then obviously there is no inherited bleeding tendency, nor any adverse reaction to anaesthesia. With regard to anaesthesia, it is important not to give repeated

halothane at short intervals, as this may produce liver inflammation (halothane hepatitis).

A history of previous operations or hospital admissions may provide clues in relation to various mouth problems and define the dental treatment required in each case.

INFECTIONS AND INFECTIOUS DISEASES

Infections may be transmitted to other patients, dentist, DSA, or other staff by cross-infections (*Figs. 4.5 & 4.6*). They may also be indicative of a disease that affects dental treatment in a different way; for example, patients with hepatitis may also have a bleeding tendency and suffer from inability to excrete drugs properly.

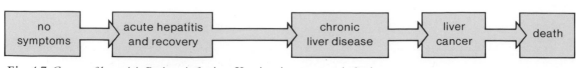

Fig. 4.7 Course of hepatitis B virus infection. Vaccination prevents infection.

Infections most likely to be transmitted in the dental surgery are respiratory (for example, common cold), or blood-borne (for example, hepatitis). Transmission is prevented by a high standard of cleanliness at all times, avoiding injury from 'sharps', avoiding contact with blood, and using disinfectants for cleaning all working surfaces. Disposable equipment is preferable whenever possible, and an autoclave is used for instrument sterilisation. Remember that dangerous infections are always a possibility; not all cases of hepatitis or AIDS have been identified.

Hepatitis

Hepatitis means inflammation of the liver, often caused by viruses. Hepatitis A virus infection is common in children, transmitted from faeces to mouth by poor hygiene. Apart from causing sickness, jaundice, itching, dark urine and pale faeces, it is a fairly harmless infection. Hepatitis A is not usually a problem in dentistry.

Hepatitis B virus infection is, however, a serious problem, as it can be transmitted by blood (for example, traces on inadequately sterilised dental equipment). It causes an illness similar to hepatitis A, sometimes combined with further very serious complications such as liver disease, liver cancer or premature death (*Fig. 4.7*). The incubation period can be up to six months. Some patients fail to overcome the hepatitis B virus and become infectious 'carriers'. Hepatitis B infection is most likely to be present in certain 'high risk' groups, and in particular:

- Patients with acute hepatitis
- Homosexuals
- Drug addicts
- Persons having spent some time in the Third World
- Institutionalised, mentally handicapped patients
- Some haemophiliacs

Transmission of the virus to dental surgery staff is most likely if the latter come into very close contact with blood, or saliva containing blood, by accidentally cutting or inoculating themselves with a contaminated sharp instrument. Transmission to patients is most likely if inadequately sterilised and infected sharp instruments are used. Transmission is, therefore, prevented by carefully disposing of such instruments (for example, needles), and using the precautions outlined in Figure 4.5. This is especially important when treating 'high risk' patients in general, or patients whose blood tests show that they are 'antigen positive' (hepatitis B antigen, or surface antigen positive). Dental staff should also protect themselves by vaccination against hepatitis B early on in their career, and have boosters every five years.

Hepatitis C and delta infections are caused by other viruses, and most characteristics of hepatitis B apply. These infections are becoming increasingly problematical in drug addicts.

HIV INFECTION AND AIDS

The acquired immune deficiency syndrome (AIDS) is an infection caused by viruses that damage certain white blood cells (T lymphocytes) and brain cells, hence the term 'human immunodeficiency virus' or HIV.

Damage to the white cells reduces the body's immunity to other infections and tumours. Therefore, patients infected with HIV may also be infected with other viruses, bacteria, fungi and parasites. HIV infection progresses to AIDS, and eventual death. HIV infection, although affecting heterosexuals increasingly, is most likely in certain 'high risk' groups including mainly:

- Homosexual or bisexual males
- Drugs addicts
- Some haemophiliacs
- Some sexual contacts of above, or persons from Central Africa

Infection is detected by a blood test for HIV antibodies, in the presence of which the test is usually positive.

AIDS may cause oral lesions (such as thrush) and tumours (particularly a cancer known as Kaposi's sarcoma), as well as enlarged lymph nodes in the neck.

HIV is found in saliva, but transmission is through blood and blood products, or by sexual intercourse. The infectivity appears to be less than that of hepatitis B virus, and incubation may spread over several years.

In the dental surgery, transmission of HIV can be prevented in the same way as hepatitis B virus, and precautions during dental treatment should be similar. So far only *very few* dental staff or patients have contracted HIV infection associated with dentistry. However, no vaccine against HIV is available at present. It must be borne in mind that patients with hepatitis may also be infected with HIV and vice versa.

JAUNDICE AND LIVER DISEASE

Jaundice is usually, but not always, caused by liver or gall stone disease. Normally, dead red cells are broken down in the liver, and their red pigment (haemoglobin) is changed to a yellow pigment (bilirubin) which is excreted in the bile. Bilirubin is changed to other pigments which colour the urine and faeces. Blockage of the bile ducts (for example, hepatitis) stops the bilirubin from being excreted in the faeces which become pale. The bilirubin accumulates in the blood and causes jaundice (yellow colour), most noticeable in the eyeballs. Its excretion in the urine in large amounts turns the urine into a dark brown colour.

The liver is an important organ, especially in the filtration and excretion of body metabolites (waste products) as well as of some drugs. It also synthesises various proteins, including some of the factors needed for normal blood clotting. Liver disease may, therefore, lead to a bleeding tendency, inability to excrete drugs (especially important in relation to general anaesthesia) and, in viral hepatitis, an infective risk.

KIDNEY DISEASE

Because the kidneys are responsible for the excretion of certain drugs, these may need to be given in a reduced dose. Patients with severe kidney disease may need kidney transplants (renal allografts). The immune system of such patients is suppressed by various drugs (corticosteroids, azathioprine, cyclosporin), and in the case of renal dialysis there used to be an increased risk of hepatitis B infection. There may also be a bleeding tendency. A few patients have gingival hyperplasia caused by cyclosporin (Fig. 9.7).

LIKELIHOOD OF PREGNANCY

Pregnancy is divided into three trimesters. During the first trimester, organs such as the heart and eyes begin to develop. During the second and third trimesters the fetus continues to develop, but growth is the main feature. Consequently, any damage to the fetus during the first trimester (for example, by infections or drugs) may lead to spontaneous abortion or to developmental defects, including brain damage. It is best, therefore, to defer dental treatment, particularly if general anaesthesia is needed, until the second trimester. At any time it is important to avoid, or reduce to a minimum, the use of drugs and radiographs. Certain drugs are absolutely contraindicated. Tetracyclines, for instance, cause tooth discoloration in the fetus or child, if given to pregnant mothers or mothers who are breastfeeding. For the same reason, they should not be given to any child before the age of eight years.

Pregnancy does not lead to an increase in caries, but patients are more liable to develop gingivitis (pregnancy gingivitis) if their oral hygiene is not thorough (page 96).

5. Diseases of the Teeth

DENTAL CARIES

Dental caries is commonly known as tooth decay. It is found worldwide, but more frequently in developed countries where sugar and other refined carbohydrates are consumed in greater quantities. The disease is caused by bacteria which are normally present even in the healthy oral cavity, in the form of plaque (page 94). It tends to be more active in children and in exposed roots, as in older patients. Enamel caries is white and chalky, but may become darker as it collects stain. Carious dentine is soft and rubbery, and ranges from light yellow to dark brown in colour. Caries spreads more rapidly in dentine than in enamel, and may undermine the enamel, giving it a bluish-white appearance. Untreated caries in dentine increasingly irritates the pulp, initially causing inflammation (pulpitis) and later possible killing part or all of it. (*Toothache* is described in the next chapter).

Areas of teeth where caries is most likely to occur are:

1. The occlusal (biting) surfaces of posterior teeth. The fissures of these surfaces trap plaque, resulting in carious cavities commonly seen in young patients. This is largely avoidable if the fissures are sealed with composite resin shortly after tooth eruption.

2. The interstitial surfaces (between the teeth), which are prone to plaque stagnation. Interstitial caries usually occurs later than occlusal caries, and in its early stages may only be detected by bitewing radiographs. Dental floss is the most efficient way of removing interstitial plaque.

Caries may also develop on other tooth surfaces, if plaque is allowed to accumulate. However, it may be reduced or even prevented if the following rules are applied (*see also Chapter 7*).

Dietary control: Reducing the amount and frequency of sugar and refined carbohydrates.

Oral hygiene: Careful daily cleaning of the teeth, to reduce plaque stagnation.

Fluoridation: Unless naturally present, fluoride may be added to the water supply by the local authority up to a level of 1 part per million. When fluoride levels in the natural or treated water supply are low, individuals may increase their intake by fluoride tablets or drops (see page 75).

Fluoride toothpaste.

OTHER CAUSES OF TOOTH LOSS

Erosion

Tooth loss may be caused by persistent contact with acid, for example, hydrochloric acid from repeated vomiting or regurgitation of stomach juices, citric acid from diets high in citrus fruit, and inhaled acid vapours from industrial processes.

Abrasion

Enamel and dentine may be worn away by being excessively rubbed with a hard object or abrasive material. Vigorous brushing with a hard brush and toothpaste will cause excessive wear of the tooth, most noticeable at the gingival margin where the enamel is thin. The enamel is soon worn away, exposing the much softer dentine which is susceptible to formation of an abrasion cavity. These cavities may be very sensitive to hot, cold and sweet substances. Treatment may consist of one or more of the following procedures:

Application of a desensitising agent, for example fluoride varnish or glycerin.

Changing the brushing method used.

Use of a soft toothbrush and low-abrasive toothpaste.

Covering the dentine with a filling, for example a glass ionomer cement.

Treat with a laser. (Lasers are a highly intensified light source which can be used via special handpieces to treat painlessly certain dental and oral problems. When in use, dental personnel and patient must wear specific eyewear. Any suction tips in use must be made of plastic.)

Removal of the pulp in severe, persistent cases.

Attrition

Loss of tooth on the biting surfaces is caused by opposing teeth wearing against each other. Some degree of attrition may be considered normal, but in excess it results in short, 'stumpy' teeth.

TOOTH CONSERVATION

The aims of restoring teeth are to prevent further advance of the carious cavity, and to return the tooth to its original shape, which ideally restores function and appearance.

Rubber dam is sometimes used to isolate a tooth during the removal of caries and placement of a restoration. This is a specially prepared thin sheet of rubber. Using a special punch, a hole is made for the tooth to poke through whilst the dam is stretched on a frame and retained on the tooth by a clamp and sometimes a ligature. The dam keeps the tooth dry and prevents contamination of the cavity. It also prevents instruments and materials from falling into the mouth. Good suction is needed to prevent a build-up of saliva behind the dam. (Rubber dam is also used to isolate a tooth during root canal treatment: page 70.)

Classification of tooth cavities

Depending on its position within the tooth, a cavity may be classified as follows:

Class I

This occurs on the occlusal surfaces of premolars and molars (*Fig. 5.1*).

Class II

This occurs at the interstitial contact points of premolars and molars (*Fig. 5.2a*). If the caries occurs only at the contact point, it may be possible to limit the size of cavity (*Fig. 5.2a*). However, combined interstitial and occlusal caries needs a mesio-occlusal (MO) (*Fig. 5.2b*) or a disto-occlusal (DO) filling. In the case of combined mesial and distal caries, the filling will be mesio-occlusal-distal (MOD).

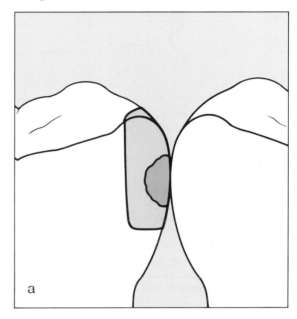

a

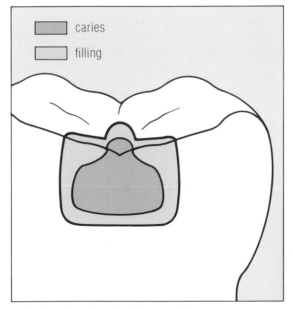

Fig. 5.1 *Class 1 occlusal caries; filling.*

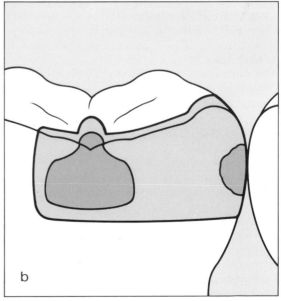

b

Fig. 5.2 a & b *Class II interstitial caries and filling; filling of mesio-occlusal cavity.*

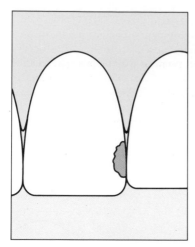

Fig. 5.3 *Class III cavity at the contact point of first and second incisors.*

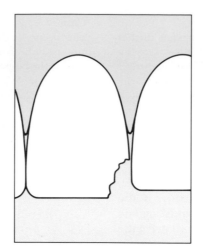

Fig. 5.4 *Class IV cavity at the incisal tip of an incisor.*

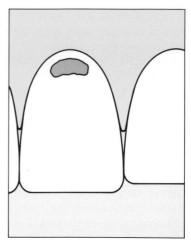

Fig. 5.5 *Class V cavity close to the gingival margin.*

Class III

This occurs where adjacent anterior teeth (incisors and canines) make contact. The cavity is normally reached by drilling from the palatal aspect. After caries removal, the cavity is hollowed out slightly, to create an undercut which will prevent the filling from falling out (*Fig. 5.3*).

Class IV

The cavity is similar to class III, but it also involves the incisal tip of the tooth (*Fig. 5.4*).

Class V

This cavity is found on the smooth surfaces of teeth, other than interstitially, and is usually close to the gingival margin (*Fig. 5.5*).

MATERIALS USED IN TOOTH RESTORATION

The most frequently used filling materials include silver amalgam, composite resin (tooth-coloured), glass ionomer cements (tooth-coloured) and gold.

Silver amalgam

This has been in use for over a century, and consists of two parts: a) silver/tin alloy in powder form, and b) mercury. The alloy and mercury are mixed together (triturated), to form the amalgam. Mixing may be done by hand (in a pestle-and-mortar), in an amalgamator where mercury and alloy are dispensed, or in a capsule where alloy and mercury are premeasured.

Mercury hazard:

Mercury, and particularly its vapour, can be poisonous if absorbed by the body even in small doses over a period of time. Therefore, every effort should be made to avoid spillage or contact with the skin. It should be stored in a cool cupboard, away from warm areas (radiators and autoclaves). Waste amalgam should be stored in an airtight plastic or unbreakable glass container with sufficient 2% potassium permanganate (or water) to cover the contents. Gloves should be worn when handling mercury or amalgam.

If mercury is spilt:

- Inform the Dental Surgeon immediately
- Ventilate the room well
- Put on face mask and rubber gloves
- Carefully scrape beads of mercury into a polythene bag for disposal
- Do NOT try to pick up spilt mercury with a vacuum cleaner
- Dispose of any contaminated soft furnishings or carpet
- Mix equal amounts of flowers of sulphur and calcium hydroxide with water and brush the creamy mix over the contaminated area; leave to dry for one to two days
- Carefully brush up the dry powder and dispose of before applying a second mix
- Repeat until all visible traces of mercury have gone

- Consult the Environmental Health Department for advice on the disposal of contaminated material
- Consult the Health and Safety Office for advice on testing the contaminated area for mercury vapour

Note that small traces of flowers of sulphur in the surgery may affect the setting reaction of silicone elastomer impression materials.

Composite resins

These are tooth-coloured filling materials, made from a clear resin and filler particles. Materials used in the past could not withstand the wear when used for posterior teeth, hence their use was restricted mainly to anterior teeth. Newer materials are now made specifically for posterior teeth, incorporating ceramic particles to improve wear resistance.

Composite resin can be bonded to the tooth enamel, which improves retention of the filling and strengthens the final product. This is done by cleaning the enamel with pumice and water, and then applying fifty percent phosphoric acid to the enamel margins for one minute. Thorough washing and drying leaves the treated enamel with a chalky appearance, and the composite resin bonds to this roughened enamel surface. This technique is known as 'acid etch bonding'. Composite resin may be bonded to dentine, using a bonding agent between the dentine and composite. Composite resin may be in the form of:

Powder and liquid.

Two-paste system where one paste contains the catalyst.

One-paste system, light-cured; this contains the catalyst which is activated only by bright light.

Glass ionomer cement

This adhesive filling material is tooth-coloured but rather opaque. It is brittle, and is therefore not suitable for the biting surfaces of posterior teeth in adults, but can be used in unretentive cavities because the cement adheres to the exposed dentine. It is slow-setting, and should be covered with petroleum jelly or varnish to prevent contamination with moisture until set. Also, it slowly releases fluoride which inhibits further caries.

Glass ionomer cement is particularly suitable for restoring:

- Abrasion cavities where there is a large area of exposed dentine, but little or no mechanical retention in the cavity.

- Cavities in deciduous teeth; because there is little need to provide mechanical retention for glass ionomer cement, cavity preparation may be kept to a minimum.

Finely ground silver particles may be incorporated within the glass ionomer to strengthen the material. The resultant cement is grey and is therefore unsuitable where there is a cosmetic consideration.

Amalgam restoration
Lay-up (with patient's records)
1. Topical anaesthesic
2. Cartridge syringe for local anaesthetic (Fig.12.1)
3. Local anaesthetic needle and cartridge
4. Dental handpieces with the appropriate burs
5. Aspirator tips and saliva ejectors
6. Gingival margin trimmers
7. Briault probe
8. PF10 lining applicator
9. Excavators and flat plastic
10. Amalgam plugger and Baldwin's burnisher
11. Ball-ended burnisher
12. Wards wax carver
13. Siqveland matrix retainers and bands
14. Wooden wedges
15. Dental napkins
16. Waste receiver
17. Cotton wool rolls and pellets
18. Lining (calcium hydroxide or proprietary forms)
19. Base (zinc oxyphosphate cement or proprietary forms), glass slab and mixing spatula
20. Amalgamator and amalgam capsules
21. Mortar and amalgam carrier
22. Pot with lid, filled with potassium permangante or water for waste amalgam

Gold

Gold has been used as a dental filling material for centuries, and is still used for inlays and crowns. An inlay is a filling cast to the shape of the cavity in the dental laboratory. The completed inlay is then cemented into the tooth cavity. Gold is, however, relatively expensive, in both material and labour costs.

Linings

Materials used as linings include calcium hydroxide, zinc oxide and eugenol, and cavity varnish. The lining is placed on the dentine inside the cavity, to protect the vital pulp against chemical irritation from the filling. It also provides some thermal insulation. Calcium hydroxide will slowly sterilise the dentine, inhibiting caries recurrence under the filling and encouraging the pulp to form secondary dentine. Zinc oxide and eugenol lining has a sedative effect on the pulp, but has none of the other advantages of calcium hydroxide.

Cements

Cements may be used in order to fill out the base of deep cavities, block out undercuts in inlay and crown preparations, cement inlays, crowns and bridges, and seal root canals. The various types of cement include zinc oxide and eugenol, polycarboxylate, zinc phosphate and glass ionomer.

CROWNS

A tooth may be crowned to restore its function and appearance if broken down, or alter the shape or position of a crown. A crown is a shell or veneer cemented on the previously trimmed-down tooth. It may be made from the following materials:

1. **Acrylic:** This is not commonly used, as it wears down and discolours with time. It is also an irritant if it comes in contact with the gum margin.

2. **Porcelain:** Hard, wear-resistant but brittle, with good stable colours. It is used mainly for front teeth, where the biting load is not excessive (porcelain jacket crowns: PJC).

3. **Gold:** Traditional, and strong when in thin sections. The edges of the gold crown, if thin, can be smoothed down by hand. As gold is soft enough to wear slightly against the opposite tooth, damage to the root is reduced. It is, however, seldom used for front teeth, for cosmetic reasons; full gold crowns (FGC) for posterior teeth are more common.

4. **Gold or nickel alloy with porcelain surface:** This crown combines the strength of gold with the good appearance of porcelain, and may be used on any tooth. It is known as a porcelain-bonded crown (PBC).

Where a tooth has a vital pulp and sufficient of the natural crown remaining (*Fig. 5.6a*), a core is prepared in the dentine (*Fig. 5.6b*). This is slightly tapered and has a smooth shoulder following the contours of the gingival margin. An impression of this as well as of the surrounding teeth is taken, from which the dental technician can manufacture the crown using any of the previously mentioned materials. This is subsequently cemented onto the core (*Fig. 5.6c*)

Where a tooth is root-filled or severely broken down, a post-crown may be indicated. If the tooth is not already root-filled, this procedure should be undertaken first (*Fig. 5.7a*). The remaining canal is widened, and a metal ready-formed or custom-made post and core cemented into it. The protruding metal core is then treated in the same way as the vital core, and a crown is constructed that fits onto it (*Fig. 5.7b*).

Jacket crown preparation and impression
Lay-up (with patient's records)
1. Topical anaesthetic
2. Local anaesthetic cartridge syringe, needle and cartridge (Fig. 12.1)
3. Dental handpieces and appropriate burs, discs, stones
4. Saliva ejectors and aspirator tips
5. Excavators
6. Flat plastic
7. Wards wax carver
8. Mitchell's trimmer
9. Scissors
10. Aspirator tip
11. Cotton wool rolls and pellets
12. Dental napkins
13. Waste receiver
14. Gingival retraction cord, solution
15. Alginate: powder, measures, water (21°C), flexible mixing bowl, mixing spatula, damp dental napkin, plastic bag, laboratory card, impression trays, fixative
16. Red sheet wax
17. Impression material: Rubber base: base and catalyst, mixing pad, mixing spatula, fixative, impression trays; Copper ring and composition: copper rings, green stick composition, spirit lamp and matches, bee-bee scissors, vaseline
18. Temporary crown forms and cement
19. Mixing pad and spatula
20. Shade guide
21. Articulating paper

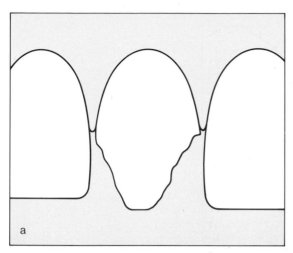

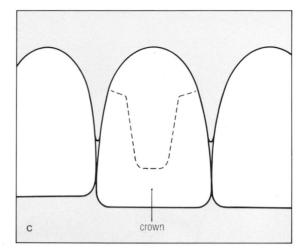

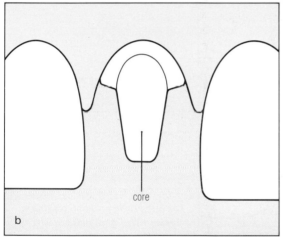

Fig. 5.6a, b & c *Broken down tooth; preparation of core; crown fitted onto the core.*

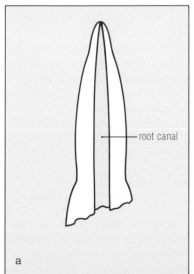

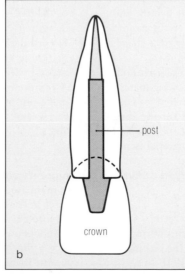

Fig. 5.7a & b *Root filling in a severely broken down tooth; new crown fitted to metal post and core in prepared root canal (see Chapter 6).*

65

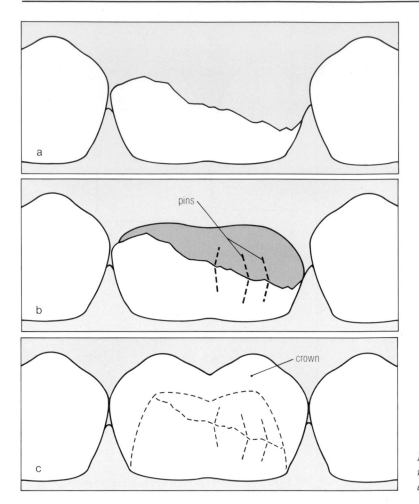

Fig. 5.8a, b & c *Broken down molar; preparation of amalgam core; crown fitted onto reduced core.*

The core of a broken down tooth may be built up by screwing small metal pins into the dentine and packing either amalgam or composite resin around them. This can then trimmed to the correct shape, and a crown is constructed (*Fig. 5.8a, b, c*).

An accurate impression of the core and surrounding teeth is taken, using one of the following materials: a) elastomer, b) reversible hydrocolloid, c) copper ring filled with hot composition for the core impression, plus alginate impression of the core and adjacent teeth. Alginate impression material is not considered accurate enough on its own.

Before the patient leaves the surgery, the following procedures are necessary:

- Alginate impression of the opposing teeth.
- Bite registration: the patient bites into warm wax or similar material, which is sent to the technician along with the other impressions. With this, the technician is able to assess the patient's dental occlusion, which is an important factor when designing a crown.
- Record the shade of the adjacent natural teeth for matching the colour of the crown. This is not necessary if the crown is to be made of gold.
- A temporary crown is constructed: this may be made out of aluminium, silver-tin alloy, or one of the several tooth-coloured plastic materials available.

Temporary crowns
The main functions of a temporary crown are to protect and cover exposed dentine (which would otherwise be very sensitive), restore tooth function and appearance, prevent the prepared tooth from overerupting or drifting, and prevent the surrounding gum from collapsing over the margins of the

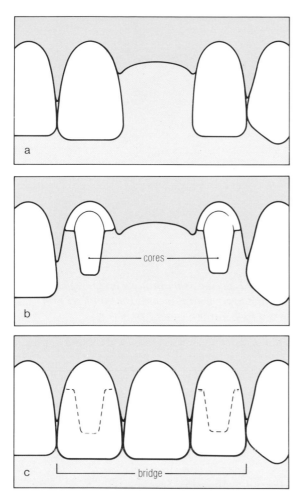

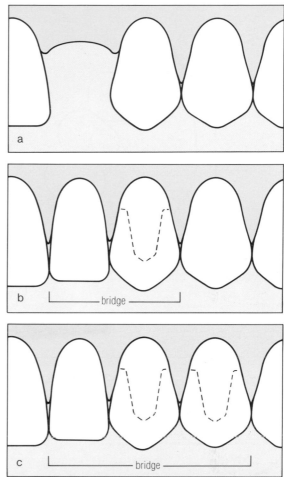

Fig. 5.9a, b & c Bridge for a missing incisor; preparation of parallel cores to serve as bridge abutments; bridge cemented into place.

Fig. 5.10 (a) Replacing a missing maxillary lateral incisor with (b) a cantilever bridge or (c) utilising double abutments on the canine and first premolar.

prepared tooth. The temporary crown is cemented in place, with a weak cement which allows its subsequent removal.

Porcelain veneers

These are very fine facings which can be cemented to the front of the teeth using acid-etched composite cement. They are constructed in the laboratory from models of the patient's teeth, and can be used to alter the colour and shape of the teeth without resorting to crowning. Veneers preserve the tooth structure and are less costly than crowning.

Bleaching of discoloured teeth is discussed on page 71.

BRIDGES

Fixed bridge

A fixed bridge is a method of replacing one or more missing teeth (*Fig. 5.9a*) with a false tooth or teeth (pontic) permanently attached to the natural teeth. In a simple fixed bridge, the teeth on each side of the space are prepared as for crowns. These are known as 'abutment' teeth and their cores should be prepared parallel to each other (*Fig. 5.9b*), with the false tooth (pontic) joined between them. The bridge is then cemented in place (*Fig. 5.9c*).

Cantilever bridge

In its simplest form, the false tooth is attached to a natural tooth on one side only (*Fig. 5.10a*). This

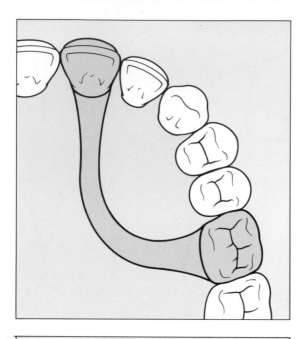

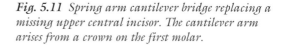

Fig. 5.11 *Spring arm cantilever bridge replacing a missing upper central incisor. The cantilever arm arises from a crown on the first molar.*

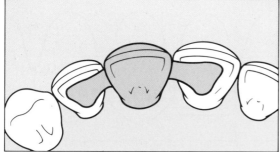

Fig. 5.12 *'Maryland' bridge.*

should only be done when the supporting abutment tooth is relatively large, firm, with a substantial root, and where the pontic space is small; for example, an upper canine abutment supporting a lateral incisor pontic (*Fig. 5.10b*). If more support for the pontic is needed, double abutments may be used (*Fig. 5.10c*). However, this design is thought to have certain disadvantages.

Spring arm cantilever bridge
The abutment tooth is some distance from the pontic, but joined to it by a metal arm; for example, an upper central incisor pontic joined across the palate to a crown on the first molar (*Fig. 5.11*). The arm is not rigid, but gains its stability from resting on the palate. Bridges of this design are no longer popular.

'Maryland' (or Rochette bridge)
This is a popular design requiring little or no preparation of the teeth on each side of the pontic (*Fig. 5.12*). The false tooth is made from metal with porcelain bonded onto the front, and from each side of the metal backing a 'wing' extends, which is secured behind the adjacent teeth using composite resin against acid-etched enamel. This design has the advantages of being quick and simple, relatively inexpensive, reversible and undamaging to sound teeth.

Special attention should be drawn to cleaning beneath any bridge, in order to keep the gums and teeth healthy. Floss cannot be passed between the teeth, as they are joined together. It should be threaded beneath the pontic, using floss threader or special floss

Implants are described on page 151.

Endodontics is the branch of dentistry concerned with the diagnosis and treatment of pulp disease and related problems.

DENTAL PULP

The pulp occupies the chamber in the centre of the tooth and consists of nerve fibres, connective tissues, blood vessels, lymph vessels and odontoblasts.

Odontoblast cells line the pulp chamber and have fine processes projecting into the dentine. Throughout life, odontoblasts generate new dentine inside the pulp chamber, called 'secondary' dentine. The process may be accelerated by low-grade irritation to the pulp, such as from a deep restoration, or from excessive tooth brushing that wears away the dentine at the neck of the tooth. When bacteria reach the pulp in large numbers, the pulp becomes inflamed.

Pulpitis

Inflammation of the pulp results in chronic low-grade pain or acute severe throbbing pain, depending on the degree of inflammation. Pulpitis may be induced by bacteria inside a deep cavity, chemical irritation from a filling placed in an unlined cavity, thermal irritation via a deep cavity, or exposed root surfaces (for example, following toothbrush abrasion), and mechanical injury to the tooth. Deep cavity preparation may, unintentionally, sometimes expose the pulp.

Chronic pulpitis

This is usually accompanied by a low-grade toothache, and may be successfully treated by removing the cause in most cases.

Acute pulpitis

This is accompanied by severe, intermittent throbbing toothache. The patient may not be able to identify the offending tooth which is usually insensitive to pressure. Pain often worsens with changes of temperature, and analgesics (pain killers) have little effect. The condition is usually treated by removal of the pulp and root canal therapy, or extraction of the tooth.

Apical periodontitis

This is inflammation of the periodontal membrane at the tip of the root. It may result from direct injury to a vital or non-vital tooth causing bruising of the periodontal membrane, or from bacteria and their chemical toxins escaping from the root canal of an infected non-vital tooth or from deep periodontal pockets. The condition may present in the form of tenderness of the tooth on biting or pressure. Pain, which does not usually worsen with changes of temperature, may range from mild to severe. Treatment consists of the following procedures:

In the case of a vital tooth with apical bruising, by removing the cause (for example, grinding down a new filling which had not been carved sufficiently to clear the opposite tooth on biting).

In the case of a non-vital infected tooth, either by root canal therapy to remove the bacteria and seal up the canal, or extraction.

Apical abscess

This is a collection of pus forming at the apex of the root. It may be chronic with only mild symptoms, perhaps with pus discharging from a hole (sinus) in the gingiva over the root, or acute with severe pain, tenderness and facial swelling. The patient with an acute abscess may feel ill, with a raised body temperature and swollen lymph nodes in the neck and under the mandible.

Chronic apical abscesses may be treated by root canal therapy. Acute apical abscesses will require drainage of pus, using the following methods:

Through an incision in the gingiva overlying the abscess.

Via the root canal.

By extraction. Systemic antibiotics may also be indicated. Once the symptoms have settled, the tooth (if still present) may be root-filled. The effects and management of these conditions are discussed further in Chapter 11.

Vitality tests
Lay-up (with patient's records)
1. Cotton wool rolls and pellets
2. Dental napkins
3. Ethyl chloride spray
4. Stick of gutta percha
5. Spirit lamp and matches
6. Electric pulp tester
7. X-ray request forms

ROOT CANAL THERAPY

The aim of root canal therapy (RCT) is to remove the pulp or pulpal remnants, clean and disinfect the root canal, and seal it with a root filling. This prevents infection of the adjacent bone.

Root canal therapy is indicated:

> In a vital tooth where the pulp is acutely inflamed (acute pulpitis).
>
> When the pulp is removed (pulpectomy), to free a large part of the root canal and use a metal post to provide support for a crown in a broken down tooth.
>
> In a non-vital tooth where the necrotic (dead) pulp is still present and likely to cause pathology at the root apex.

Access to the pulp chamber is obtained through the crown. In premolars and molars this is achieved via the occlusal surface, while in incisors and canines it is usual to approach via the palatal (upper) and lingual surfaces (lower).

Root canal treatment
Lay-up (with patient's records)
1. Rubber dam sheet, punch, clamp, clamp holders, frame
2. Dental floss
3. Excavators
4. Flat plastic
5. Lateral condensers
6. Spirit lamp and matches
7. Scissors, ruler
8. Selection of reamers and files
9. Rubber stops
10. Barbed and smooth broaches in holders
11. Rotary paste fillers
12. Paper points
13. Cotton wool pellets and rolls
14. Waste receiver
15. Reamer cleaner
16. Saliva ejector
17. Aspirator tips
18. Dental handpieces and appropriate burs
19. Local anaesthetic cartridge syringe, needle and cartridge
20. Topical anaesthetic
21. Gutta percha and silver points
22. Disposable 2ml syringe and needle for irrigation
23. Saline and root canal sealant
24. Glass slab and mixing spatula
25. Permanent filling material or temporary dressing

Safety chains should be fastened to the handles of reamers and files as a safeguard against their being swallowed. However, teeth undergoing root canal therapy are usually isolated with rubber dam, as described on page 61.

Once the pulp chamber is reached, the pulp is removed (extirpated) using either a barbed broach (fine wire with barbs along its length), or a reamer. A radiograph is taken with the reamer inserted into the root canal to the estimated length of the tooth (diagnostic film). From this radiograph the tooth length may be calculated reasonably accurately. The 'working length' is the length of the tooth minus a millimetre or two, to ensure that the filling is placed inside the root and does not pass beyond the root apex. The canal is finally cleaned to the working length with progressively larger reamers or files, until it is clean and smooth. Engine-driven reamers are available which may reduce operator fatigue. Root canals may also be cleaned ultrasonically.

If the canal has previously been infected, it is advisable to wash it out using a sterile saline solution, or sodium hypochlorite solution. The canal is dried using sterile paper points and the access cavity sealed with cotton wool and a temporary cement filling; a small amount of disinfectant solution (for example, camphorated monochlorophenol) may be added to the cotton wool. At the next appointment the canal is sealed, provided there is no indication of persistent infection.

Where there is no initial infection of the canal it is possible to complete the therapy in only one visit using:
- A silver point plus cement.
- One or more gutta percha points plus cement.
- Cement on its own.
- Amalgam.

Pulp treatment for children is described on page 78.

APICECTOMY
This is a surgical method of removing apical infection and placing a root canal seal directly at the end of the root. It is indicated when root canal treatment cannot be carried out satisfactorily, for example:

- In a very curved root.
- Where a root filling has already failed and a second attempt is impossible (for example when a metal post has been cemented into the canal to support a crown).
- Where the canal is too narrow to allow the passage of even very fine reamers.

- When root filling material has passed through the apex into the surrounding bone and is acting as an irritant.
- When the end of the root has been fractured following an injury, and needs to be removed.
- When an apical infection will not respond to normal root canal therapy.

Access to the root apex is obtained via a flap made in the mucosa overlying the tooth. This may be performed under local or general anaesthesia. Alveolar bone over the root apex is removed with a bur in a straight handpiece, with water irrigation. Once the root apex is located, the top is flattened and a small retentive cavity made in the canal opening. The amalgam, or gutta percha, or zinc oxide and eugenol cement is introduced into the cavity to seal it. The operation is completed by cleaning the wound and closing the flap using sutures. Patients should expect some pain and swelling after apicectomy, and advice similar to that following a dental extraction must be given (page 146).

BLEACHING

In certain circumstances discoloured natural teeth may be lightened using bleaching agents.

For root-filled teeth these may be applied within the tooth, *via* the access cavity of the root filling. The tooth must be isolated with rubber dam (page 61), and the patient's eyes, face, and clothing should all be protected from any splashes. The usual bleaching agent is 30 per cent aqueous hydrogen peroxide.

Vital teeth may be bleached by applying a less caustic bleaching agent to the outer surface of the teeth on a daily basis for several weeks. This technique is usually considered suitable for home use.

Any improvement in colour following bleaching is not normally permanent, and from time to time the procedure may need repeating.

7. Children and Dentistry

Children need to be given special consideration in the dental surgery. The DSA should always try to speak to them so that the face is at the same level as the child's. This is best achieved by bending at the knees. Smiling and speaking gently and clearly in a language that will be understood helps to establish a good first impression of the dental environment.

Small children should be led by the hand into the surgery; it may also be helpful to hold the child's hand during examination and treatment. Parents are not encouraged to come into the surgery, unless the child is very small, or the parent's presence is requested by the dentist. The following points should be remembered:

- It is useful to have a fair amount of comics and books in the waiting room, as well as posters on the walls at a suitable eye level.
- It must be checked that the child taken into the surgery is the one expected by the dentist, and not a brother or sister instead.
- Promises that cannot be fulfiled, for instance, 'it won't hurt', are to be avoided, as they may cause disappointment and mistrust.
- A routine visit to the lavatory is a sensible precaution.
- Only a small proportion of children are truly difficult, and experience should enable the DSA to understand and handle them as necessary.
- Children become more anxious than usual if they have to wait a long time. Therefore, suitable appointments must be made for them, preferably not at the end of a busy day.
- Some children are frightened, others are difficult, and some are both: a frightened child needs reassurance, a sympathetic manner, careful explanation of what the dental visit involves, and awareness of the cause of fear. Fear may be objective, following previous experience (for example, a traumatic general anaesthetic or toothache), or subjective, having heard exaggerated stories concerning dentists and treatment. In either case, the parent should be helpful. Sometimes, however, the parent communicates fear to the child, probably unintentionally.

On the other hand, a difficult child needs firm yet sympathetic handling. If the parent is excluded from the surgery, this often removes the 'showing off' syndrome. Assessment of these children is the dentist's responsibility, although making certain that the dentist is prepared for the case beforehand can be of great help. The amount of treatment for a difficult child will depend upon each individual response. It may be that only a prophylaxis is carried out at a first visit, or nothing at all.

> **It must be remembered that dentistry can, and should, be fun for children.**

IN THE SURGERY

Dental equipment can be fascinating or terrifying to small children. To the dental team the surgery is an everyday place of work; to the small child it is an alien environment. Therefore, all essential instruments visible to the child must be kept to a minimum; mirror, probe and tweezers should suffice initially. 'Injection' is understood by most school-children, but terms such as 'needle', 'drill' and 'hurt' are better avoided. Strong lights into children's eyes are also to be avoided, as are sudden movements, particularly in relation to tipping the chair back. Even coming too close to the child may cause fear. Most children are ticklish, and 'tickling' a tooth with a brush, rubber cup or even a bur can have some children laughing merrily.

Modern dental chairs will accommodate children well. Where the headrest is removable, it should be removed if the child's head does not reach it. Also, check that children are seated comfortably, as they have a tendency to slide so that their chin rests on their chest, which makes proper dental examination impossible.

The DSA may talk to the child if the dentist is talking to the parent, but should not distract the dentist. Very small children may be more easily examined when lying on their mother's lap. Treatment for them can be carried out with their head on the dentist's lap, or in the crook of the mother's arm.

Children sometimes cry. Babies cry when uncomfortable or hungry, toddlers when frustrated or unhappy, or when they have hurt themselves: the mother can usually discern the reason. In the surgery, small children may be genuinely upset. Older children may have found that crying is a means of avoiding something, perhaps an injection. Firm handling may be necessary ('shut up and sit still' technique), but a more gradual introduction is usually more appropriate ('tell, show, do, praise' technique). Generally, a gentle approach works well with small children.

CHILDREN'S TEETH

Babies are normally born without teeth. Occasionally a tooth may be present at birth, but this is usually lost as no root has yet formed. Such a tooth would also interfere with breastfeeding.

The first deciduous ('milk') teeth to erupt are usually the lower central incisors, at about six months of age. The upper central incisors follow soon afterwards; the lateral incisors erupt at nine months, the first molars at twelve months, the canines at eighteen months, and the second molars at twenty-four months. There are five deciduous teeth in each quadrant (total of twenty, see page XX). There are no deciduous premolars. The eruption chronology given is based on normal averages (*Fig. 7.1*). Therefore delayed or early eruption between three and six months should not be considered abnormal.

Teething may be completely trouble-free, decidedly unpleasant, or anything in-between. Parents often seek advice: gels containing a local anaesthetic for rubbing into the gums and various 'teething' toys can usually give relief. If the child refuses to eat, analgesics may be prescribed for taking half-to-one hour before meals (see also page 119).

TOOTH	AGE
Central incisor	6 months
Lateral incisor	9 months
Canine	18 months
First molar	12 months
Second molar	24 months

Fig. 7.1 Average ages at which deciduous teeth erupt. Note that there are no deciduous premolars and that lower teeth usually erupt before uppers.

Deciduous teeth

Deciduous teeth are smaller, whiter and more bulbous than permanent teeth. The deciduous molars have less enamel and dentine in proportion to pulp, and with the pulp horns reaching deeply into the cusps. The first molars (Ds) have a unique crown form and do not resemble any permanent teeth. The second molars (Es) resemble the first permanent molars in crown form, number of cusps (four for the upper and five for the lower), fissures and shape. They also have the same number of roots (three for the upper and two for the lower). The roots are widely divergent, and the premolars develop between them. The incisors and canines resemble permanent teeth in shape and number of roots (one root each).

Permanent teeth

Permanent teeth generally erupt without problems. However, if the gingiva overlying an erupting lower molar is traumatised by the already erupted upper tooth (see page 101 and *Fig. 9.14*), it will create a painful and self-perpetuating condition unless treated. Treatment consists of reducing inflammation, usually with a hot saline mouthwash, and keeping under observation. Occasionally, it is necessary to excise the gum flap. Parents sometimes notice a bluish swelling over an erupting tooth: this is an eruption cyst which will disappear as the tooth erupts.

The first permanent tooth to erupt is usually the first molar, followed by the lower central incisor. This happens around six years of age; parents frequently do not realise that the extra tooth at the back of the mouth is a permanent tooth. Permanent lower incisors often erupt lingually to the deciduous incisors and sometimes form two rows of teeth. Unless the deciduous incisors show no sign of being lost, no treatment is necessary.

Permanent teeth are yellower than deciduous teeth, and parents often ask about 'yellow teeth': this usually calls for reassurance, but the dentist should be consulted. Newly erupted teeth are more likely to become carious than teeth that have erupted for a year or more.

As the deciduous teeth are shed and replaced by permanent teeth, the child enters the 'mixed dentition' stage. Girls generally lose their deciduous teeth earlier than boys. There is a wide variation in the ages at which teeth are lost and replaced; the average ages for eruption of permanent teeth are shown in *Fig. 7.2*.

TOOTH	UPPER	LOWER
Central incisor	7 years	6 years
Lateral incisor	8 years	6/7 years
Canine	11 years	9 years
First premolar	10 years	10 years
Second premolar	11 years	11 years
First molar	6 years	6 years
Second molar	12 years	12 years
Third molar	15+ years	15+ years

Fig. 7.2 Average ages at which permanent teeth erupt.

PREVENTIVE DENTISTRY

If it is possible to cultivate good habits early on in life, then the risk of dental disease can be minimised throughout life.

Dental health education
The aims of dental health education are to minimise dental caries, instil good tooth cleaning habits so that periodontal disease is minimised in later years, and make people aware of the importance of teeth and supporting structures.

Dietary advice
It is unreasonable to expect patients to adopt an entirely non-cariogenic diet immediately and clean their teeth meticulously. However, it is necessary to get children and parents to accept the idea that the process of disease can, indeed, be prevented if dental advice is followed, and then to act upon that advice. The DSA may, under instructions from the dentist, offer dental health advice to parents and children. The messages should be brief and accurate:

- Nearly all mouths contain the type of bacteria which cause tooth decay.
- It is not possible to eliminate these bacteria on a long-term basis.
- Bacterial plaque (see Chapter 9) will collect on the teeth and gums whether we eat or not.
- Many foods contain simple sugars which bacteria convert to acids; these acids remove minerals (calcium salts) from the tooth enamel. This is how caries starts.
- Sugars (refined carbohydrates) are present in virtually all tinned foods (especially fruit), biscuits, fruit drinks, jams and confectionery, and are an integral part of our daily diet.
- Teeth can remineralise from calcium salts that exist in saliva. Therefore, saliva can replace lost calcium salts maintaining a calcium balance. This, however, can only occur if the saliva is given adequate time to work on the teeth: restriction of sugar to main meals only ensures that any calcium loss can be replaced.
- If in-between meal snacks are unavoidable, then those not containing sugar are preferable (crisps, nuts, selected fruit).
- There are three essential ingredients for caries: teeth, bacteria and refined carbohydrates. If one is eliminated, no caries results. The easiest to eliminate is the refined carbohydrate.
- Parents should be told of the dangers of using sweetened dummies, propped feeding bottles and undiluted vitamin syrups.

An enthusiastic approach will often encourage both children and adults. Children respond well to approval and praise, adults more to social conformity; if mothers were told that ninety-five percent of parents brush their children's teeth, they might start doing so themselves, which would help achieve this currently mythical figure.

Oral hygiene instruction

The DSA, as well as the dental hygienist and dental therapist, can given oral hygiene instruction under the direction of a dentist. It is important that what is being taught is up-to-date and in accordance with the dentist's wishes.

Toothbrushing

Toothbrushing can never remove bacterial plaque from all fissures or interproximal areas where teeth are in contact. However, this does not mean that it is useless, as it certainly assists in the prevention of cervical cavities and other smooth surface lesions. Children under seven years of age cannot clean their own teeth effectively, and must by supervised by parents who should complete the process of tooth cleaning for them. It does not matter if the child chews the brush at first. Parents should stand behind the child in front of a mirror, so that both can see what toothbrushing involves. In any case, the technique is less important than the result. Disclosing agents may be used; if supplied for home use, the parents must be instructed adequately. Floss, although very effective, is not generally recommended for children; adults must be instructed on how to use it properly.

Cleaning should start when the first teeth erupt, and the first toothbrush may well be a cotton bud. Deciduous teeth have a self-cleansing shape and are relatively easy to clean. However, plaque must still be removed, and regular thorough brushing should become a habit built up from the earliest days. A fluoride toothpaste must always be used, but without overloading the brush, as children tend to swallow rather than rinse out.

The ideal toothbrush should have a small head with two or three rows of multi-tufted soft, nylon bristles. The handle should be straight, quite short and broad, so that small hands can hold it easily. When the bristles become permanently deformed, usually after about two months' use, the brush should be replaced.

Fibrous foods, such as carrots, celery and apples, have little effect on tooth cleaning, but are otherwise beneficial.

Fluoride treatment

This is classified into systemic and topical:

Systemic
Water supply
Fluoride tablets and drops
Salt, bread, milk
Toothpaste

Topical
Toothpaste
Gels and solutions
Rinses
Varnishes

Fluorine is an element, similar to chlorine and iodine, which has a strong inhibitory effect on dental caries. Fluoride is a salt that contains fluorine, and acts in several ways:

It reacts with enamel to make the enamel crystals more resistant to acid attacks.

It helps in the process of remineralisation of enamel where the latter has already been attacked, making better crystals when these are precipitated in the presence of fluoride ions.

It is absorbed by bacteria in plaque, where it blocks their reaction with sugar, thus preventing them from producing acids too readily.

Systemic fluoride

If fluoride is present in the diet during the years that the crowns of the permanent teeth are forming (namely, from birth to twelve years), the full thickness of enamel is fluoridated. The crystal structure is improved, becoming more compact, and the teeth tend to be slightly smaller, with more rounded cusps and shallower fissures.

The best and most effective way of ensuring an adequate intake of fluoride is through the waste supply. There is always some fluoride in the water and, in certain areas only, it reaches the concentration of one part per million (1ppm) which has been shown to given the maximum benefit in caries prevention without mottling of permanent teeth. Fluoridation is the adjustment of the amount of fluoride to 1ppm.

Fluoride tablets or drops have exactly the same effect and achieve the same caries control if taken consistently from six months. The tablets may be sucked or chewed; there are arguments as to which is most beneficial, but in either case they need to be

DAILY DOSAGE OF FLUORIDE				
Fluoride concentration in water supply	Age (years)			
	0–1/2	1/2–2	2–4	4+
<0.3ppm	—	0.25mg	0.50mg	1.00mg
<0.7ppm	—	—	0.25mg	0.25mg
>0.7ppm	—	—	—	—

Fig. 7.3 *Daily dosage of fluoride in relation to the child's age and the concentration of fluoride in the water supply.*

pleasantly flavoured. Drops are added to drinks of small infants. Dosage is reduced if the amount of fluoride in the water supply is between 0.3–0.7ppm. No extra fluoride should be given if the concentration in the waste exceeds 0.7ppm (*Fig. 7.3*). Fluoride tablets and drops are now prescribable under NHS regulations in Britain.

Tablets should be kept in a safe place away from children. Fluoride can also be added to salt, bread and milk, with beneficial effects. Most toothpaste sold in Britain contains fluoride in some form. It was originally thought that this had a purely topical effect but, while for adults this is probably so, it gives children a boost to their systemic intake, as they have a distinct tendency to eat it.

Topical fluoride

Fluoride ions permeate the outer layers of the enamel and enter the crystals of calcium hydroxyapatite of which the enamel is composed. The ions are chemically bound and change the chemical and physical characteristics of the enamel.

Fluoride toothpaste containing 0.8% sodium monofluorophosphate, sodium fluoride (in some cases both) or stannous fluoride, constitutes ninety-eight percent of the toothpaste market. This is a most convenient and frequent method of applying fluoride to the outer layers of tooth enamel, because of the number of topical applications. The effect is greatest on newly erupted teeth, as the surfaces of unerupted teeth are porous and only mineralise fully when exposed to calcium salts in saliva. Hence the presence of fluoride ions favours mineralisation of this porous surface zone. Fluoride toothpaste saves approximately one new surface from becoming decayed each year compared with unfluoridated

toothpaste, so that over the period of eruption of the permanent dentition the cumulative effect is quite considerable. In caries-prone children it may be advisable to discourage rinsing out after brushing with a fluoride toothpaste: a residual film of toothpaste remaining over the teeth, particularly where trapped in carious cavities, allows continuing fluoridation.

Fluoride gels and solutions contain acidulated phosphate fluoride (APF) consisting of 1.23% fluoride ions. These flavoured gels may be applied directly to the teeth with a cotton bud, quadrant by quadrant or, alternatively, to the entire dental arches in one application by inserting 'trays' into the mouth: specially constructed foam or trays are partly filled with gel and inserted into the mouth over the dental arch for four to five minutes. A saliva ejector is essential.

Prior to applying the gel or solution, the teeth should be cleaned with a non-fluoride, non-oily, prophylactic paste or pumice. Interdental plaque is removed with dental floss and thoroughly dried with the air syringe, to prevent dilution of the gel by saliva. After removing the tray, excess gel is wiped off the teeth so that it is not swallowed. The patient should not eat or drink for thirty minutes after treatment.

The solutions and gels are highly concentrated. A 250ml bottle of gel contains three lethal doses for a 20kg child.

Flavoured gels or solutions must never be left within reach of small children when unattended.

To be effective, gels must be applied regularly by the dentist, therapist or hygienist. The frequency of application depends upon the requirements of the individual patient, but usually takes place every four months.

In caries-prone children, sodium fluoride mouth rinses are prescribed (0.05% solution for daily use, 0.2% solution for weekly rinses or for use in organised schemes in schools). The solution should be forced through the interdental spaces to act on the interstitial surfaces; a quantity of 5–10ml of solution is held in the mouth for one minute, but must not be swallowed.

Varnishes are sticky, resinous fluoride substances, painted onto cleaned, dried, enamel surfaces of teeth. Although the varnish dissolves away slowly, it remains in contact with the enamel for a sufficiently long time to have beneficial action.

There also are several prophylactic pastes which contain a high proportion of fluoride; therefore care must be taken not to swallow paste.

It must be noted that too much fluoride can lead to mottling (white spots) on teeth, but it has been shown that there is more mottling in non-fluoridated than in fluoridated areas. Water fluoridation is still the best and most economical method of ensuring sufficient fluoride intake.

Fissure sealants

A clear or tinted layer of resin is applied to the etched occlusal surfaces of molars and premolars to reduce fissure caries. Teeth are dried and cleaned, using a non-fluoride, non-oily paste. They are then isolated, either with rubber dam or cotton wool rolls. High volume aspiration and/or saliva ejector are essential. An etching solution or gel, usually containing thirty percent phosphoric acid, is applied for at least 30 seconds and each tooth is washed with water for at least 15 to 20 seconds. The dried tooth should appear chalky: if not, etching is repeated. If etching is satisfactory, a sealant is applied (one drop of resin and one drop of catalyst mixed together, placed on the tooth and allowed to set for a few minutes). Alternatively, the sealant may be painted onto the tooth and light cured.

If done properly, the efficacy of this treatment is extremely good; where, however, isolation is poor or saliva contaminates the etched surfaces, sealant adhesion will also be poor.

Conservation of children's teeth

The materials used are the same as those used for adults: amalgam, composite, glass ionomer and occasionally gold. Stainless steel, porcelain and gold may be used for crowns.

Amalgam

Instrumentation is the same as for adult treatment:

- Records and radiographs
- Mirror, probe and tweezers
- Pluggers
- Carvers
- Matrix bands
- Handpieces and burs
- Local analgesia, as required

Deciduous teeth, because of their bulbous shape, require wedges for accurate adaptation of matrix bands around interstitial cavities.

Composite

Similar instruments are required as for amalgam, but pluggers should be made of plastic and matrices of nylon or celluloid. If light-cured composites are used, then patient, operator and DSA should all have eye protection. Composites are best used with acid-etch techniques: because etchant contains thirty percent phosphoric acid, care should be taken that spillages do not burn clothes and/or skin. Deciduous teeth may need increased etching time (two minutes is advised). Acid should not be applied directly to dentine: lining must be applied first. Composites should not be lined with zinc oxide/eugenol materials, as eugenol reacts with the resins in composite.

If a molar or premolar has a small cavity, the dentist may undertake a 'sealant restoration' (or 'preventive resin restoration'). This involves a mixture of composite in a small cavity and fissure sealant over the entire occlusal surface. This is performed in stages:

1. Cavity preparation
2. Lining
3. Etching
4. Placement of composite restoration
5. Placement of fissure sealant

Glass ionomers

Instrumentation is similar to composites; plastic instruments are not particularly important. This treatment is used increasingly in children, especially for deciduous teeth. It contains fluoride which is slowly released, hopefully preventing further caries. It is mixed to a thick paste according to manufacturers' instructions, and will adhere to dentine. Lining, except in very deep cavities, is not needed. There should be protection with varnish or petroleum jelly after setting, and the inside surfaces of matrix bands should be coated with a thin layer of petroleum jelly before placement.

Like composites, glass ionomers should not be placed over zinc oxide/eugenol materials.All these materials are best used under rubber dam; clamps are available for deciduous molars.

Stainless steel crowns

Badly broken down, but saveable, deciduous teeth (as well as first permanent molars) may be restored with stainless steel crowns. Caries must be removed and the tooth reduced all around, to enable fitting of the crown: the occlusal height is reduced and all carious lesions are blocked out. The tooth is then measured mesiodistally, and an appropriate pre-formed crown is selected. The crown is trimmed with Beebee crown and collar shears, and fitted to the tooth so that a snap fit is obtained. Contouring pliers are required for this purpose. The crown is finally removed from the tooth, dried, and then cemented in place. Care is required while handling the crowns during trimming; the cut edges tend to be very sharp.

Pulp treatment for children

Blood supply to the pulp in children is usually good, as the apices of permanent teeth are wider than in adults. Deciduous teeth have tortuous and often multiple root canals, which makes conventional root canal treatment virtually impossible. Small exposures of the pulp in both deciduous and permanent teeth may be capped with a calcium hydroxide material. The prognosis in permanent teeth is usually good, but in deciduous teeth it is variable. Larger exposures require pulpotomy, namely, partial removal of the pulp. Pulpotomy for permanent teeth (usually incisors) involves the following procedures:

- Local anaesthesia and rubber dam.
- Entry to pulp chamber obtained through the palatal aspect with wide extension.
- Coronal pulp removal with a sterile excavator.
- When bleeding ceases, remaining pulp is covered with calcium hydroxide and quick-setting zinc oxide/eugenol.
- Radiograph is taken.
- After regular checks over a period of three to four months further radiographs are needed to check the apex (whether it continues to close up) and the root canal (formation of barrier in response to calcium hydroxide).
- If satisfactory, the tooth is reviewed until root

formation and apical closure are complete. Further review concerns possible full endodontic treatment (see pages 69–70), with or without definitive restoration of the crown.

In deciduous teeth, pulpotomy may be either vital or non-vital, and usually involves the molars.

Vital pulpotomy

In vital pulpotomy the pulp is exposed during cavity preparation.

One-stage treatment: Under local anaesthetic, the pulp chamber is opened and the coronal pulp removed. Formocresol is applied to bleeding remnants for four minutes (CARE: this substance will burn if spilt on the gingiva). The cavity is then washed with normal saline, sterile water or local anaesthetic. This procedure is repeated until bleeding stops. Next, quick-setting zinc oxide/eugenol containing one drop formocresol is applied; a cement base is inserted and the tooth restored with amalgam or stainless steel crown.

Two-stage treatment: If not under local anaesthetic, the exposure should be opened as widely as possible and caries removed; paraformaldehyde paste is applied to the exposure and sealed with quick-setting zinc oxide/eugenol. The patient should be warned of possible pain for the initial few hours. The tooth is reviewed after two to three weeks, or as necessary. It should then be reopened, washed and pulp remnants removed. The procedure may require repeating until the pulp is completely non-vital.

Mortal (non-vital) pulpotomy

The affected tooth usually has a discharging sinus, usually buccally, but it may be lingually. The tooth is normally painless and the condition is often unnoticed by the parent. Abscess formation in deciduous teeth is usually interradicular, at the bi- or trifurcation of the roots. The floor of the pulp chamber is very close to this area, which means that the dentine is thin.

The tooth is isolated, preferably with rubber dam (page 61), and the pulp chamber opened. If the tooth is abscessed, this means that the tooth is non-vital and the procedure should be painless. Any pulp remnants are removed and the chamber is cleaned; a drop of beechwood creosote on a cotton wool pledget is placed in the cavity (CARE: this substance will burn if spilt on the gingiva), with a dressing of quick-setting zinc oxide/eugenol. This is left for two weeks and the tooth is then isolated, re-opened and the pulp chamber is washed. The procedure that follows is the same as for vital pulpotomy. Any sinus should disappear after a few weeks. Periodic radiographs will show whether healing is taking place.

Pulpotomy in deciduous teeth is successful in about seventy to eighty percent of cases. It is performed in order to keep the dentition intact, avoiding balancing extractions, and to maintain space for the permanent dentition. Where teeth are spaced, crowding of permanent teeth is less likely and extractions may be considered as an alternative.

Open apex treatment

Occasionally, a permanent tooth does not respond to pulpotomy, or the patient is not treated after an accident until the pulp has died. Root canal treatment of an incompletely formed root can cause problems.

The tooth is isolated, preferably with rubber dam. The root canal is located, and good access to the canal is obtained. It is then reamed and filed as necessary. A radiograph is taken to determine the working length; calcium hydroxide is spun into the root canal, using a spiral filler (Lentulo spiral), and another radiograph is taken. Regular radiographs are needed until bony resolution has occurred. Repeated calcium hydroxide dressings may also be required. The root canal is then washed clean and filled with gutta percha points condensed together to seal the canal, and a final radiograph is taken.

Trauma

Most everyday accidents do not affect children's teeth, but some do. Deciduous incisors are those most commonly affected, and may appear either dark brown to black or opaquely cream. If dark, bleeding has taken place inside the root canal and pulp chamber, indicating that the tooth is non-vital; if opaque, calcification of the pulp chamber has taken place, and the tooth may or may not still be vital. In either case, reassurance is all that is necessary. A few cases will develop buccal swellings, with or without pain (usually painless). If the tooth is not exfoliated at the correct time, the permanent teeth may be delayed or erupt in the wrong place: extraction is normally required in these cases.

Very rarely, the permanent tooth may be affected and 'dilacerated', that is to say, the crown and/or root are bent, in which case the permanent tooth may not erupt. Deciduous teeth may be knocked back into the gum; the vast majority of these will re-erupt naturally.

Permanent teeth tend to break; fractures may be of the enamel, for which smoothing off the rough surface is usually enough. If there is a fracture of enamel and dentine, this will require immediate attention: a radiograph is taken and the tooth isolated. The exposed dentine is covered with a calcium hydroxide cement, and the enamel is etched. The tooth is then covered with a composite. Vitality should be checked several weeks later.

Fracture of enamel, dentine and pulp may require pulp capping, pulpotomy or pulpectomy, depending on the severity of damage and the patient's age. Fracture of the root may require splinting or extraction, depending on the site and severity of damage. Sometimes no treatment is required. Accidents can also cause displacement of teeth, and even total loss. If displaced, a minor displacement may be left alone where the occlusion is not affected. Major displacements may be realigned and splinted, until healing of the surrounding tissues occurs.

Teeth can be replanted if seen soon enough; the best way to preserve the tooth until it reaches the surgery is in the patient's or parent's saliva or, alternatively, in milk. The periodontal membrane should be left as intact as possible (and *not* scrubbed) and the tooth repositioned in the mouth as soon as possible. Splinting will be required until initial healing takes place. Roots of replanted teeth tend to resorb: root filling with calcium hydroxide helps to keep this under control.

PREVENTION OF ACCIDENTS TO TEETH

Children participating in contact sports should wear a properly fitting mouthguard. Mouthguards are quickly and easily made in PVC, following a routine upper alginate impression

'DIFFICULT' AND HANDICAPPED CHILDREN

Some children, for a variety of reasons, find the acceptance of dental treatment difficult. Some are frightened, and really need reassurance and tender loving care, coupled with a slow introduction to dental procedures. Others are simply unable to accept treatment in the routine way; they may have physical and/or mental handicaps, or they may simply be 'difficult' children. Inhalation sedation (Relative Analgesia; see page 134) can given a reasonable degree of relaxation (sufficient to enable a spastic patient to relax and be able to control spasms) but will only work, like most other means of sedation, if the patient co-operates. Some handicapped children, for instance many Down's syndrome cases, can be managed in the normal surgery, but other will require reference to specialist hospital facilities.

79

8. Orthodontics

Orthodontics is the branch of dentistry concerned with the treatment of irregularities in the articulation of teeth and jaws known as 'malocclusion'.

Approximately sixty percent of children have a degree of malocclusion sufficient to warrant treatment. Apart from the obvious cosmetic advantages of well aligned teeth, orthodontic treatment can play an important role in the prevention of dental disease: dental articulations may be harmful to the teeth or their supporting bone, resulting in excessive tooth wear (attrition), or damage to the gums and mandibular joints. These problems can be easily avoided by timely orthodontic treatment in early childhood.

Although adults may benefit from orthodontic treatment, this usually tends to be part of tooth repair; in order, for example, to allow placement of periodontal splinting, or to permit fitting of bridgework.

Orthodontic treatment is usually carried out in the early teens, when most of the permanent teeth have erupted but the patient is still growing rapidly. This is desirable because the bony changes necessary to tooth movement occur more readily in growing children. In addition, as orthodontic treatment carried out in childhood is likely to modify facial development, it is necessary for the orthodontist to have a detailed understanding of this development, in order to estimate any changes that may occur in the individual patient and plan the appropriate treatment to the patient's advantage.

CLASSIFICATION OF OCCLUSION AND MALOCCLUSION

In an ideal dental occlusion, the sixteen teeth in each arch form a regular curve; the dental arch and all thirty-two teeth are accommodated without any overlapping. In addition, every tooth of the upper jaw should occlude with (bite against) of the corresponding tooth of the lower arch and the tooth posterior (distal) to it (*Fig. 8.1*). This is because the upper central incisor is much wider than its lower counterpart; the cusps of the upper canines, premolars and molars fit into the appropriate fossae of the lower teeth and vice versa. However, an ideal occlusion is extremely rare in Britain.

The first molars are among the teeth of the permanent dentition that erupt early on, thus giving an indication of future occlusion. It was this initial occlusion on which Edward Angle, an American pioneer of modern orthodontics, based his classification of malocclusion. Unfortunately, the first permanent molars are sometimes lost due to dental decay, and frequently drift forwards in the arch when deciduous teeth have been lost prematurely. Therefore, most orthodontists prefer to classify malocclusion according to the way the incisors meet, known as the 'incisor classification'. The molar occlusion is recorded separately.

Class I
This type of malocclusion occurs in about fifty percent of the English population. The relationship of

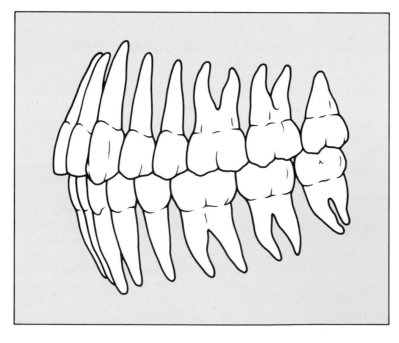

Fig. 8.1 Normal (ideal) dental occlusion.

the two arches is correct, therefore incisors and molars meet properly; that is to say, the lower incisor edges contact the middle of the palatal surface of the upper incisors, and the mesiobuccal cusp of the upper first permanent molar occludes with the buccal groove of the lower. It is still possible for some of the teeth to be in incorrect positions, for example the jaws may be overcrowded, but the general 'front to back' articulation of the teeth is correct (*Fig. 8.2*).

Class II

This type of malocclusion occurs in about forty-five percent of the population: the upper arch is too proclined (or the lower is articulated too far back), and the molar occlusion usually reflects this arrangement. Edward Angle found that the incisor teeth of Class II malocclusions fall into two categories (*Fig. 8.3*).

In Class II, division 1 (about thirty percent of the population), the front teeth are proclined; that is, tipped forward such that they often protrude between the lips. The horizontal distance between the upper and lower incisor teeth (overjet) is increased.

In Class II, division 2 (about fifteen percent of the population), the upper central incisors are tipped back into contact with the lower incisors. The overjet is therefore reduced, but the vertical overlap (overbite) is increased.

> **Overjet:** The extent to which the upper incisors project beyond the lower incisors.
>
> **Overbite:** The extent to which the upper incisors bite over the lower incisors.

Class III

This type of malocclusion occurs in about five percent of the population: the lower arch is too far forward (or the upper arch is too far back). The overjet is reduced (*Fig. 8.4a*) and the incisors may bite edge-to-edge. Sometimes the difference in arch relationship is severe enough to cause the upper incisors to fit completely inside the lower incisors, in which case the overjet is said to be 'reversed' (*Fig. 8.4b*).

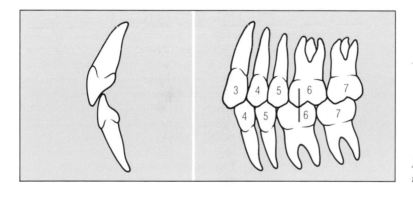

Fig. 8.2 Class I dental malocclusion.

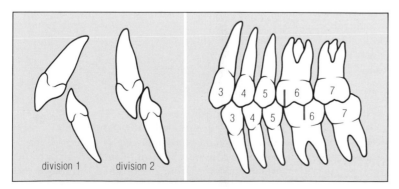

Fig. 8.3 Class II dental malocclusion; divisions 1 & 2.

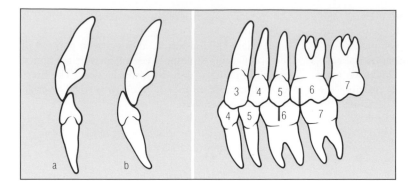

Fig. 8.4 Class III dental
malocclusion; a & b.

Crossbite

So far, dental occlusion has been considered with
the patient's dentition viewed from the side. If
viewed from the front, it will become obvious that
in an ideal Class I occlusion all the upper teeth meet
with half their crowns outside (labially or buccal to)
the lower teeth. In cases where the positions of
upper and lower teeth are reversed, the condition is
known as a 'crossbite'. This may affect only one
tooth, or all the posterior teeth on one side (unilat-
eral crossbite), or occasionally *all* the posterior teeth
(bilateral crossbite).

CAUSES OF MALOCCLUSION

Malocclusion may be produced by any one of a large
number of causes which render ideal occlusion a rare
phenomenon. Nevertheless, all factors can be fitted
into three main causative categories but, before clas-
sifying them, it would be helpful to cover in broad
terms how an ideal dentition develops.

Teeth develop within the maxilla or mandible. As
they erupt from these skeletal bases towards each
other, they are moulded by the pressure of lips and
cheeks on one side, and the tongue on the other
(soft tissues, *Fig. 8.5*). For an ideal occlusion these
bases need to be correctly related, therefore if the
lower base lies too far back with respect to the upper
it is likely that a Class 2 type of malocclusion will
develop. Conversely, a Class 3 malocclusion is more
likely to occur when the lower base lies too far forwards with respect to the upper (*Fig. 8.6*).

The forces produced by the soft tissues are very
light, but quite sufficient to move the teeth.
Generally, those forces will establish the teeth into
correct positions, but sometimes the actions of the
muscles are unusual or, in the case of thumb sucking, their normal action is impeded.

Local factors

Once the teeth erupt, the form of their biting surfaces (occlusal) together with the action of biting
(occlusal forces) gradually guide each opposing
tooth into the final relationship with its opponent.
The position of a particular tooth is also affected by
pressures from other teeth, permanent or deciduous,
in front of and behind it. Thus, removal of a tooth
while the dentition is still developing can have a
marked effect on the position of adjacent teeth,
especially if these are erupting or just about to erupt.
Such local disturbances are known as 'local factors'
in malocclusion.

Common examples of local factors are premature
extraction of deciduous teeth, supernumerary (extra)
teeth, teeth of unusual size or form, and missing
teeth (having failed to develop). Occasionally, only
one factor may be responsible for malocclusion, but
usually two or more act together. In summary, factors are grouped as follows:

1. Skeletal (relationship of facial bones)

2. Soft tissues (actions of lips, cheeks and
   tongue)

3. Tooth arch disproportion (crowding or, more
   rarely, spacing)

4. Local (such as thumb sucking, extra and
   missing teeth).

Biology of tooth movement

Bone is a living tissue and, throughout life, its constituents are constantly replaced. If an arm or leg is
broken, new bone will form in such a way as to be
indistinguishable from the original. Although the

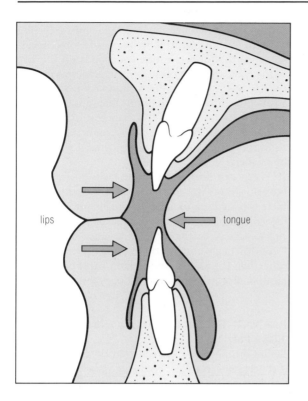

Fig. 8.5 *The lips and tongue play an important role in the formation of dental occlusion.*

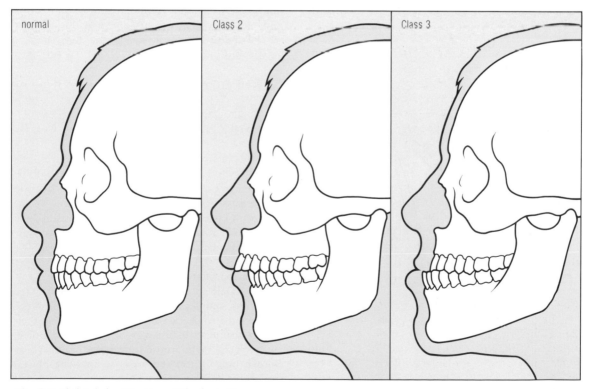

Fig. 8.6 *Skeletal classification of the dental bases.*

mechanism is not yet fully understood, it has been known for many years that bone changes its shape according to the forces acting on it. In the same way, light forces applied to the teeth cause the surrounding bone to be removed from one side of the root surface to the other. Hence the tooth moves inside the bone (*Fig. 8.7*). To be effective, these orthodontic forces must be very gentle (otherwise they damage the tooth or bone), as well as continuous. This is often not appreciated by patients who think that removing an appliance for an hour or two each day will have no effect on the treatment; in reality, it may well bring treatment to a standstill.

Even under ideal conditions, teeth move quite slowly in response to orthodontic forces, not more than a millimetre each month. It also takes time before cells which remodel the bone begin to appear. This explains why it takes about two weeks before a tooth under continuous force from an orthodontic spring starts to move. Once the teeth reach a correct position, they must be held ('retained') for several months to allow the final bony changes to occur, so that the occlusion remains stable after appliance wear is discontinued.

The degree of force is quite critical: if too small, tooth movement will not take place at the optimum speed; if too large, the root of the tooth and surrounding bone may be damaged, thus reducing the rate of movement. The degree of force necessary to orthodontic treatment depends on the size of the root, the type of movement undertaken, and the age of the patient. For a single-rooted tooth in a patient of normal orthodontic age (around twelve years), a force of 0.25–0.3 Newton (25–30g) is recommended for tipping movement. For larger teeth the force will be greater; for adults it should be smaller.

Teeth can be moved quite easily in direction, buccally, lingually, mesially or distally, provided there is bone for a tooth to be moved into. Intrusive movement (upwards into their sockets) is more difficult to achieve, as the tooth is designed to resist the forces of occlusion. Extrusive movement on the other hand must be undertaken carefully, as the tooth is effectively being pulled out of its socket.

PLANNING THE ORTHODONTIC TREATMENT

Before orthodontic treatment can be decided upon, it is necessary to collect complete information about the form of the jaws and the positions of erupted and unerupted teeth. This information is obtained from pretreatment records:

1. Plaster casts (study models) made from impressions of the teeth

2. Radiographs of the teeth and jaws

3. A radiograph of the head (cephalometric or lateral X-ray) (page 18)

In many practices, even where the dentist gives little or no orthodontic treatment, the DSA will be expected to prepare the study models and develop radiographs. For this reason, the procedures will be dealt with in some detail. It is also essential for the dentist to be aware of the patient's attitude to treatment, particularly if this involves appliance wear.

Preparation of study models

Study models are taken both at the planning stage and after completion of treatment, to allow the orthodontist to check that the teeth remain in their correct positions. Impressions are taken in alginate, using special orthodontic impression trays. A wax 'squash bite' is also required, so that the plaster models can be prepared to represent the exact dental arrangement and occlusion in the patient's mouth.

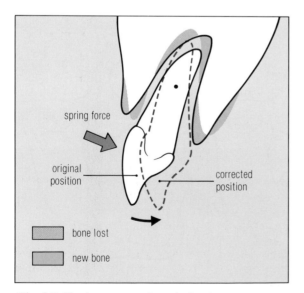

spring force

original position

corrected position

bone lost

new bone

Fig. 8.7 Tooth movement in orthodontics.

Impressions should be rinsed in cold water to remove saliva and mucus; they are then covered with damp gauze and placed, as a pair, in a polythene bag with the correct wax squash bite. They must be clearly labelled (either by tying on a label, or by writing on the border of the impression with an indelible pencil), and should be cast as soon as possible.

Models are made (cast) by pouring white plaster or yellow 'artificial stone' into the impression. The DSA will need to be shown how to do this. Once the plaster is fully set (when the model becomes hot), the impression can be carefully removed and the model trimmed using a special electric model-trimmer.

Models must be trimmed as a pair by fitting the wax squash bite over the upper and lower teeth. This must be done with care, otherwise the model may break. It is usually helpful to soften the wax slightly in warm water, to allow it to be fitted on more easily. The pair is then held against the rotating surface of the model-trimmer, so that the base and sides of the model can be ground.

Orthodontic radiographs

These must show the crowns and roots of both erupted and uncrupted teeth. Sometimes a combination of periapical and bitewing radiographs may be used. A much better picture with less radiation is obtained with special X-rays. Routine orthodontic radiographs involve either an orthopantomogram, or left and right oblique lateral views, plus a nasal occlusal X-ray of the upper incisor region. The orthopantomogram requires a special X-ray machine; the oblique lateral radiographs may be taken on a conventional dental X-ray machine, but require special cassettes to hold the film.

ORTHODONTIC APPLIANCES

Patient tends to call any orthodontic appliance a 'brace'. In the United States this means a fixed appliance cemented to the teeth, whereas in Britain it is thought of as a removable appliance worn in the upper arch. It is, therefore, best to avoid the term 'brace' in the surgery and refer to appliances as 'removable' and 'fixed', using their correct names.

Removable appliances

Teeth moved orthodontically with removable appliances will always tilt to some extent, due to the shape of the roots (see Fig. 8.7). However, provided that the teeth can be tipped into acceptable positions; a removable appliance has several advantages:

It can be put together in the laboratory, which makes it inexpensive.

It is relatively simple to adjust, requiring little clinical time.

It is safe; if troublesome, it can be removed for short periods by the patient.

It may be removed for cleaning, therefore oral hygiene is seldom a problem.

It may be removed for contact sports, therefore damage to the patient (and appliance) is reduced to a minimum.

If damaged, it can usually be repaired fairly easily, either at the dental surgery or in the laboratory. Should it be beyond repair, the appliance may be adapted so that orthodontic progress is retained whilst a new appliance is prepared.

The disadvantages are that removable appliances tend to be rather bulky and take some time to get used to. They are also unsuitable for most treatment in the lower arch, as the shape of the lower teeth does not allow the appliance to be satisfactorily retained.

The removable appliance consists of several wire components embedded in a plastic base plate which holds them together (Fig. 8.8). These elements can be grouped into two types:

Retentive: Wire clasps holding the appliance in place by gripping the crowns of teeth.

Active: Springs and screws which apply pressure to individual teeth, causing them to move.

When the appliance is supplied by the laboratory, the springs are designed to just touch the teeth without applying any force (passive). To activate a spring, the dentist will need to bend (adjust) its position so that, when the appliance is placed in the mouth, the spring gently pushes the tooth in the desired direction.

Adams clasp (crib)

This clasp has been designed for molars, for which it is almost solely used (it is sometimes seen on other teeth). Where headgear is to be used, tubes are usually soldered to Adams clasps on molars.

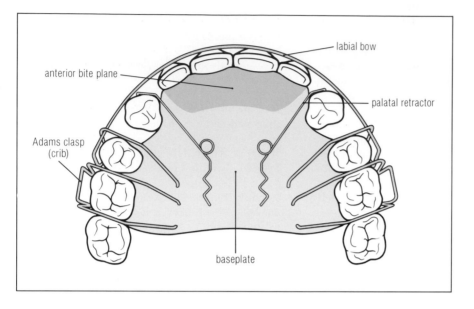

Fig. 8.8 *A maxillary removable appliance comprising springs and clasps in a plastic baseplate.*

Labial bow

This is a wire running around the front of the incisors, usually extending as far as the canines. It is used for retaining the appliance, and can also be modified to move the incisor teeth during later stages of treatment.

Roberts retractor

This is a form of labial bow but made of a thinner wire (0.4mm) than the standard labial bow (0.7mm), which makes it more flexible. It is, therefore, a rather better type of labial retractor. The disadvantage is that it is unsuitable as a retainer.

Palatal spring (finger spring, cantilever spring)

This is the commonest type of spring used for moving canines and premolars along the line of the arch (mesially or distally). It consists of a tag embedded in the baseplate, a coil and a straight section (arm) which extends from the coil to slightly beyond the point of contact with the tooth. In order to protect the spring and at the same time allow movement, the arm and coil lie in a hollow part of the fitting surface of the baseplate.

Buccal spring

This is another kind of retractor used only where the canines are displaced too far towards the cheeks (buccally). It approaches the tooth from the buccal sides (hence its name). This spring lies mainly outside the protection of the baseplate. For this reason it has to be made of the thicker wire (0.7mm), so as to resist the forces of biting.

Z-spring

As its name suggests, this has a 'Z' shape and is used for moving instanding incisors forwards into their correct position, biting outside (labial to) the lower incisors.

T-spring

This spring also takes its name from its shape. It is used for buccal movement of instanding premolars or molars.

Expansion screws

There is a variety of expansion screws, but they all work on the same principle: a threaded screw is set into a tiny metal framework; as the screw is turned, the two halves of the framework gradually slide apart. The screw is set between two parts of the acrylic baseplate of the appliance, and its action is to move one group of teeth away from the others. The screw plate is adjusted by the patient, who must remember to turn the screw with a special key a quarter of a turn each week.

Bite planes

Teeth may also be moved by forces of occlusion. The simplest and most common example in an upper removable appliance is the anterior bite plane, which is a raised area of plastic just behind the front teeth. Because the lower front teeth bite upon this platform and the posterior teeth are left free to erupt, the bite plane is used to reduce excessive incisor overbites.

Clinical procedures
Orthodontic examination
The object of the initial orthodontic examination, lasting about fifteen minutes, is to collect all relevant information about the nature and cause of the particular malocclusion. Once this is obtained, an appropriate treatment plan can be made.

Lay-up (with patient's records)
1. Mirror, probe, college tweezers
2. Stainless steel ruler (calibrated in millimetres)
3. Dividers

The examination usually takes place in the presence of the parent. Initially the patient is seated in an upright posture, whilst the dentist carries out the extraoral examination (skeletal relationship, form and behaviour of the lips). This is then followed by the intraoral examination carried out in the normal dental operating position. If not already available, routine orthodontic radiographs will be taken, and if the patient is judged to be ready for treatment, impressions will be required for preparation of study models.

Treatment planning
At second visit, lasting between fifteen and thirty minutes, the treatment procedures are decided upon and outlined to the patient and parent for their approval as regards the type of appliance required and any extractions which are necessary.

Lay-up (with patient's records)
1. Mirror, probe, college tweezers
2. Stainless steel ruler (calibrated in millimetres)
3. Dividers
4. Photographs or examples of orthodontic appliances
5. Routine orthodontic radiographs
6. Study models (trimmed)

If the patient accepts the treatment plan and is ready for treatment with removable appliances, the dentist may take further impressions (working impressions), so that the appliance may be ordered. The appliance design must be sent with the working impressions, and annotated on the patient's 'work card' (often the same card used for prosthetic and other laboratory work).

Fitting and adjustment of appliances

Lay-up (with patient's records)
1. Mirror, probe, college tweezers
2. Stainless steel ruler (calibrated in millimetres)
3. Dividers
4. Photographs or examples of orthodontic appliances
5. Routine orthodontic radiographs
6. Study models (trimmed)
7. Adams pliers, to adjust molar clasps
8. Spring forming pliers, to adjust and modify springs.
9. Wire cutters, to shorten springs
10. Wax pencil, to mark wire or baseplate
11. Straight handpiece and acrylic bur, to relieve acrylic, and thus permit tooth movement
12. Full face mirror, so that the patient can be shown how to remove and replace the appliance.

The fitting of the first appliance may require half-an-hour. Subsequent routine adjustments will not take more than fifteen minutes. The DSA may be required to give the patient and parent instructions on the wearing care of appliances. Briefly, these are:

The appliance should be worn all the time (including meal times).

It should be rinsed after meals and cleaned at least twice a day when normal toothbrushing is carried out.

The patient may experience some difficulty with eating and speaking, but this will soon pass. The teeth may also ache a little when the springs are first activated.

It is very important to seek immediate help if the appliance is uncomfortable, damaged, or broken.

Sticky foods will damage the appliance.

Where the practice is only carrying out orthodontic treatment, it is best to remind parents that the child must still see the dental practitioner for routine treatment.

It is usual to allow up to two weeks for the patient to get used to the appliance before carrying out any tooth extraction. Routine adjustments are needed every four to six weeks.

Fixed appliances

The only way to prevent a tooth tipping in response to an applied orthodontic force is to attach a channelled 'bracket' to its crown and compel the tooth to slide along an 'archwire'. Because the appliance is firmly attached to the teeth, it is referred to as 'fixed'.

Generally, attachments are required on all upper and lower teeth, This usually means that there will be brackets bonded to the incisors, canines and premolars, as well as stainless steel buccal tubes welded to molar bands and cemented to the first permanent molars. Such appliances have to be constructed in the patient's mouth and are, therefore, difficult to adjust. Fixed appliance treatment is usually confined to hospital departments and to dental practices where the practitioner has received postgraduate orthodontic training.

Fixed appliance components

There are many different types of fixed appliances. In Britain, two types are commonly used: the Edgewise appliance (*Fig. 8.9*) and the Begg appliance (*Fig. 8.10*). Each of these has its own type of bracket for anterior teeth. The molar tubes are of round cross section for the Begg appliance, but rectangular for the Edgewise technique. If headgear is required, a double molar tube will be used.

The archwires are either bent into shape at the chairside, or preshaped. In the Edgewise technique, the archwire is held in the brackets with soft, stainless steel tie wires called 'ligatures', or small plastic rings known as 'elastic modules'. In the Begg technique, the arch is pinned into place with special brass pins (Begg pins).

Teeth move by the action of archwires, and also by the force produced by the various elastic materials. Some of these run between the brackets (chained elastic modules), and others from the upper arch to the lower (intraoral latex elastics).

Clinical procedures
Orthodontic examination

This lasts approximately fifteen minutes. The purposes and instrumentation are exactly the same as for removable appliances.

Treatment planning

This lasts thirty minutes. The purpose and instrumentation are the same as for removable appliances. If treatment is to be started immediately, the orthodontist may place 'separating springs' or 'elastic separators' mesially and distally to each molar, to allow bands to be placed at the subsequent visit. Separation takes about ten minutes and the lay-up is the same as for examination, but it includes either separating springs placed with light wire pliers, or brass wire or elastic separators places with mosquito forceps.

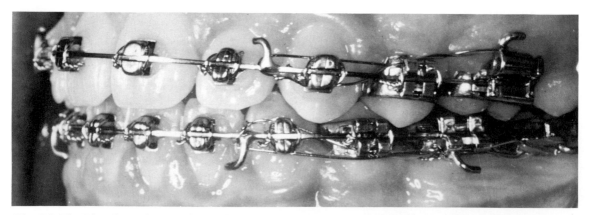

Fig. 8.9 *The Edgewise appliance. This appliance uses a rectangular archwire. This example shows 'straightwire' brackets which save the orthodontist a great deal of time since the arch used is in the form of a simple curve without any complex bends. However, for this to be possible, each bracket is slightly differently machined and so there is a different bracket for each tooth which the DSA must be able to recognise. Note that the brackets have a tiny indentifying mark on the disto-gingival wing to ensure that it is placed the right way up.*

Placing the bands

This is carried out approximately one week after separators are placed. First, the separators are removed and the contact area is cleared of any food debris; then, appropriate size bands are chosen (there is a range of sizes for both upper and lower molars), using the study models as a guide. This takes between thirty minutes to one hour.

Lay-up

1. Records, radiographs
2. Safety spectacles, protective bib
3. Mirror, probe, college tweezers
4. Cotton wool rolls and saliva ejector, to dry the tooth for cementation
5. Band pusher, to push the band down and over the tooth
6. Biting stick, to allow the patient to bite the band down into its final position.
7. Band-removing pliers, to remove the band for cementation
8. Mitchells trimmer, to remove excess cement
9. Spatula, glass or plastic flat slab, for mixing oxyphosphate or polycarboxylate cement and loading it inside the band

It is usual for anterior brackets to be bonded in place at the same appointment, using an acid-etch technique. In most practices, the instruments for bonding are kept as a bonding kit and are very much a matter of individual choice depending on the technique and bonding agent used.

Begg: placing or adjusting archwires

Archwires may be placed at the same visit as banding and bonding but, if so, the appointment will last over an hour.

Lay-up

1. Records, radiographs
2. Safety spectacles, protective bib
3. Mirror, probe, college tweezers
4. Study models
5. Wax pencil, for marking wire
6. Light wire pliers, to form or adjust the archwire
7. Howe pliers (straight), for placing Begg pins
8. Distal end cutters, for removing excess archwire projecting beyond the molar tubes
9. Wire cutters, for cutting appropriate lengths of high tensile wire for forming into arches
10. Ligature cutters, for cutting out old ligatures
11. Serrated scissors, for cutting ligature wires
12. Twiddler (ligature tucker), for tucking cut ligature wires behind the archwire so that they do not project
13. Ligature wire, Begg pins

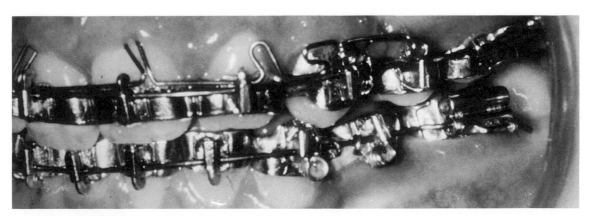

Fig. 8.10 *The Begg appliance. This uses round wires and in Stage III of the treatment shown here there are two arches, one placed on top of the other and a number of auxillary springs. Note that, in this rather old illustration, bands are used for the anterior teeth rather than bonded brackets. These days, bands are only used on anterior teeth for special reasons — for example where the tooth has already been restored using the acid-etch technique and removal of a bracket might also dislodge the restoration.*

Edgewise: placing or adjusting archwires

Lay-up

1. Records, radiographs
2. Safety spectacles, protective bib
3. Mirror, probe, college tweezers
4. Study models
5. Wax pencil, for marking wire
6. Light wire pliers, to form or adjust the arch-wire
7. Distal end cutters, for removing excess arch-wire projecting beyond the molar tubes
8. Wire cutters, for cutting appropriate lengths of high tensile wire in order to form into arches
9. Ligature-locking pliers, for placing and tying ligatures
10. Ligatures cutters, for cutting out old liga-tures
11. Serrated scissors, for cutting ligature wire
12. Twiddler (ligature tucker), for tucking cut ligature wires behind the archwire, so that they do not project
13. Preformed ligatures of a special 'hairpin' shape to fit the ligature-locking pliers
14. Mosquito forceps (2 pairs) for placing elastic modules

Headgear

Headgear may be used in conjunction with both fixed or removable appliances, and consists of an elasticated headcap or neckstrap which transmits force through a wire frame known as a 'facebow' because it looks rather like the instrument used in prosthetics to record jaw relationships. In fact, most dentists and all patients refer to this part of the headgear as 'whiskers', because from the back the patient appears to have a wire whisker coming out of each corner of the mouth. Where removable appli-ances are used, the headgear fits into a tube soldered onto the molar clasps or special hooks added to the front of the appliance. In fixed appliance treatment, it is inserted into tubes soldered onto molar bands or special loops bent into the archwire. Headgear is used to overcome the tendency of back teeth to be pulled forwards during orthodontic treatment. This is particularly important in those cases where tooth removal has provided just enough space to align the front teeth.

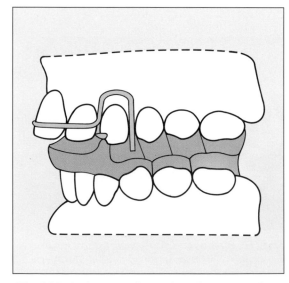

Fig. 8.11 Andresen appliance, here shown on study casts. Note the facets in the acrylic.

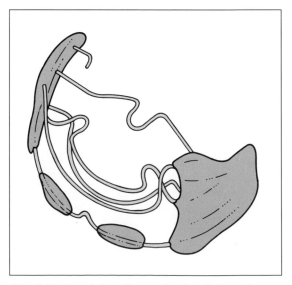

Fig. 8.12 Frankel appliance, showing the buccal shields, lip pads, and labial arch.

Instructions to patients wearing fixed orthodontic appliances

Patients should be informed that the appliance is fixed to the teeth and cannot be removed except by a dentist. It is, however, delicate and should be treated with care.

Ordinary food can be consumed, but apples should be cut up and sticky toffee must *not* be eaten.

The teeth and appliance should be cleaned with a soft toothbrush after each meal or snack, care being taken to remove food under wires.

If the appliance is damaged or bands loosen, the surgery should be contacted immediately.

When fitted, the appliance may cause some slight discomfort; with perseverance, it should pass off within 24 hours; if not the surgery should be contacted.

Regular attendance for routine dental check-ups is important

Myofunctional appliances

Another kind of appliance ought to be mentioned here, although it is, in fact, a special kind of removable appliance. As the name suggests, myofunctional appliances work by harnessing the action of facial and jaw muscles. They produce dental changes which resemble the tipping actions of removable appliances, but these may also have some influence on jaw development. The most important members of this group are called 'Andresen' (*Fig. 8.11*) and 'Frankel' (*Fig. 8.12*).

Cleft lip and palate

Treatment of orthodontic problems of patients with this condition is an important part of the hospital-based orthodontic consultant's work. It should be emphasised that the orthodontist is only one of the cleft palate team which consists of a plastic surgeon, an oral surgeon, a speech therapist and a general dental practitioner. Orthodontic treatment begins immediately after birth, when the infant requires a plate to cover the cleft and give a near-normal palate both for feeding and to encourage moulding the two halves of the cleft closer together. After repairs to the lip and/or palate are undertaken, further early treatment may be requires. Finally, there is almost always a need for a course of fixed appliance treatment at the normal orthodontic age, which sometimes involves corrective jaw surgery (orthognathic surgery).

9. Periodontology

Periodontology is the study of the periodontium (*Fig. 9.1*) and its diseases. The periodontium of each tooth is made up of:

- Gingiva (gum)
- Cementum
- Bone
- Periodontal membrane

The cementum, bone, and periodontal membrane together support the tooth. Periodontal diseases threaten that support.

THE HEALTHY PERIODONTIUM

A thin layer of cementum coats the dentine of each tooth root. Attached between the cementum and the wall of the bony socket is the delicate periodontal membrane (described on page 37). The crown enamel and root cementum of each tooth meet (sometimes incompletely) along a curving boundary called the cemento-enamel junction (CEJ), sometimes also called the amelo-cemental junction. The crest of the healthy bone socket is normally about 2mm from the CEJ of a fully-erupted tooth (*Fig. 9.2*). Between the roots of the back teeth the bone crest is rather flat and broad, but it is more ridge-shaped between the front teeth. Sometimes the bony covering of a root is incomplete because of a V-shaped defect in the bone margin (called a 'dehiscence') or a window-like defect (called a 'fenestration') in the socket wall. Also, bony enlargements sometimes occur.

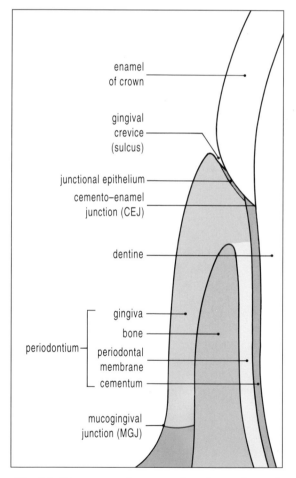

Fig. 9.1 *Diagrammatic cross-section of part of a tooth showing component parts of periodontium and related structures in health. See also Figs. 3.2 and 9.3.*

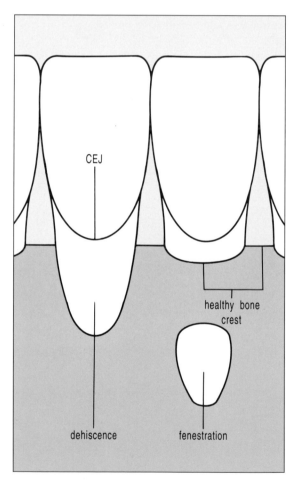

Fig. 9.2 *Lower incisor teeth showing the position of the healthy bone crest (normally about 2mm from CEJ) and two anatomical variations (dehiscence and fenestration), all normally covered by gum (see Fig. 9.3).*

The bone and that part of the crown and root of the tooth either side of the CEJ are normally covered by the gingiva (gum). In health, the gingival margin normally rises and falls around the mouth as it conforms to the undulations of the CEJ of each tooth. Filling the space between each tooth and the underlying bone crest are peaks, each called a gingival papilla (plural: papillae) (*Fig. 9.* 3), which tend to be broader between the back teeth than between the front teeth.

Healthy gingiva is pale pink, or pigmented to a varying extent, with a firm texture and a dotted (stippled) surface (*Fig. 9.4*). A change to a more reddish colour, where the gingiva meets the softer tissues reflected from inside the cheeks and lips, marks a boundary called the muco-gingival junction (MGJ) (*Fig. 9.3*). Between the central incisors prominent web-like structures, each called a frenum (plural: frena) cross between lip and gum; similar but smaller structures may be seen at other sites.

The healthy gingival margin is sharp and not enlarged. On its inner surface it is securely attached to enamel by a specialised band or cuff of tissue called the junctional epithelium, except just inside the gingival margin where there is a minute, shallow, space called the gingival crevice (or gingival sulcus) about 2mm or less in depth. Gingival (crevicular) fluid, derived from the serum, constantly passes out into the mouth *via* the junctional epithelium and crevice.

Many patients seem to regard gingival bleeding as normal. However, bleeding on toothbrushing is a sign of disease (page 95), not of health. Healthy

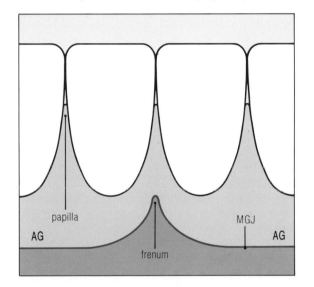

Fig. 9.3 *Features of a healthy gingiva: papilla; marginal gingiva; frenum; mucogingival junction (MGJ); attached gingiva (AG).*

HEALTH	INFLAMED (CHRONIC GINGIVITIS)
Pale pink (or pigmented)	Reddened
Firm consistency	Soft, shiny, swollen
Stippled surface	Stipples disappear
Sharp gingival margin	Blunting of papillae and margins
Not prone to bleed with toothbrushing	Prone to bleed with toothbrushing
Shallow crevice (sulcus) present	"False" pocket develops
Junctional epithelium present	Pocket epithelium forms from junctional epithelium

Fig. 9.4 *Gingiva in health and disease.*

gums should not bleed during normal toothbrushing.

Occasionally, even in health, the gum margin recedes, probably over a dehiscence, exposing part of the root; such an area of localised recession is sometimes called a Stillman's cleft (*Fig. 9.5*). Lower incisors seem most prone to this problem. The future of the affected tooth is rarely at risk, but the exposed root may be very sensitive and can look unsightly (*see also Figs. 9.30 and 9.31*).

Before continuing, you may find it helpful to identify in your own mouth the visible features described in this section.

PLAQUE

Before looking at the diseases of the periodontium, we need to say something about dental plaque, a term meaning the soft but complex layer of bacteria often found sticking to the teeth, and causing tooth decay (caries) and periodontal diseases in many individuals.

Bacteria (microbes, micro-organisms, 'germs') are found in all mouths except those of newborn babies. They also inhabit other parts of the body. They are minute, self-contained, units of many different types. Although each consists of a single cell, sizes vary. In

shape, some are round, others are like rods (straight or curved), commas, threads, or spirals. Some move; others do not. Most are either 'Gram-positive' or 'Gram-negative' depending on their reaction to the special Gram's stain used in microbiology. In addition, various bacteria thrive only in the presence of oxygen (referred to as being 'aerobic') although some require only a minimal amount; others (referred to as being 'anaerobic') thrive only in the absence of oxygen (which is toxic to them); others can adapt to the presence or absence of oxygen, and yet others require carbon dioxide for growth ('capnophilic').

How does plaque form? A completely clean tooth surface is soon covered by a thin film ('pellicle') of salivary material. Single aerobic Gram-positive bacteria soon adhere to this film and begin to multiply, spreading across the tooth as early plaque and being joined by other bacteria. Unless this process is halted by cleaning the tooth, plaque becomes thicker and more extensive. The inevitable reduction in available oxygen, and production of carbon dioxide, favours the growth of bacteria suited to these changes. Plaque also includes substances produced by these bacteria, which may in turn encourage the growth of other bacteria. It also may include food particles, although plaque is not the same as food residue and, unlike food particles, cannot be removed by eating fibrous foods or rinsing. Early plaque is invisible, but later becomes visible to the trained eye, and can be shown up ('disclosed') by certain dyes. In time it may partially harden to form calculus ('tartar') (page 103), and both may later become stained by tar (from smoking), tea, coffee, and other dietary substances.

It is important to realise that, even in the same mouth, plaque in different sites may be composed of different bacteria. In some areas, plaque growth may constantly be limited by tooth cleansing, but in inaccessible sites plaque growth and development may continue unhindered. As the potential for causing disease is partly governed by the presence of certain bacteria and the substances which they produce, different levels of disease may be found in the same mouth. The *amount* of plaque at a site is no indicator of its ability to cause disease. As we shall see later, this is particularly true of periodontal diseases.

Plaque and caries

As explained earlier (page 60) enamel caries is less common on smooth tooth surfaces than in fissures and between the teeth on approximal surfaces. The micro-organisms most closely associated with the

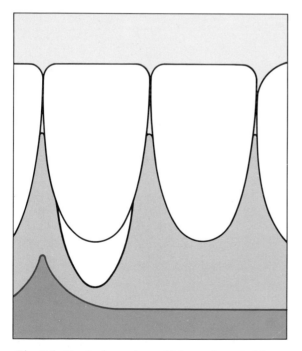

Fig. 9.5 Gingival recession, which may be caused by vigorous, incorrect toothbrushing, but probably overlying a dehiscence.

onset of caries at these sites are members of the *Streptococcus mutans* group, which are round cells, with a tendency to form chains, which are Gram-positive and aerobic. Basically, from sucrose in the diet they form an acid able to attack enamel; repeated presentation of sucrose (such as in frequent sugary snacks) can therefore cause persistent enamel attack which in time leads to caries. Other microorganisms are of course associated with caries, particularly a Gram-positive rod called *Lactobacillus* which requires minimal oxygen for growth.

In some individuals, caries can develop in roots exposed by gingival recession (see *Figs. 9.5, 9.13 and 9.31*).

GINGIVITIS

Gingivitis means gingival inflammation.

Plaque tends to collect particularly between the teeth and at the gum margin (*see Fig. 9.1,* page 92), thereby reaching the inside of the crevice. Bacterial products enter the adjacent tissues, provoking an attempt by the body to overcome them by the process of inflammation: the blood flow at the site increases and fluid enters the tissues, bringing — in increasing numbers — a sequence of specialised defence cells and protective substances to the area. In this way, the body's immune response gets under way. Some of the defence cells appear in the increased flow of crevicular fluid, and special methods now exist for examining substances in this fluid.

These changes start to affect the appearance of previously healthy gingiva after a few days. Where plaque is accumulating, the papillae and marginal gingiva gradually become swollen (rounded or blunted), soft, shiny ('glassy') and red; the stipples disappear (*Fig. 9.4*).

At the same time the structure of the tissues gradually alters. This involves the junctional epithelium which starts to lose its tight attachment to the enamel, so forming a space between the inflamed gum and enamel which in reality appears to be a deepening of the original crevice. This space, formed as a result of disease, is called a *pocket* (*Fig. 9.6*) (more precisely, a 'false pocket' or 'pseudo-pocket', to distinguish it from a 'true pocket' as found in periodontitis; page 96). The altered, diseased, junctional epithelium which lines it is called, not surprisingly, 'pocket epithelium'.

The bacteria which initiate the sequence of changes just described are basically those found in health, so their ability to cause disease results from their greater numbers as a consequence of inadequate tooth cleaning. This early plaque is dominated by Gram-positive aerobic *Streptococci*. However, thread-like bacteria soon appear in the undisturbed plaque, and the utilisation of available oxygen then begins to favour the growth of anaerobic forms and other bacteria with more stringent requirements.

Bacteria, of course, readily accumulate on the enamel inside the pocket, where they are eventually beyond the reach of a toothbrush and remote from saliva with its antibacterial properties. Bacteria in the pocket favour the progression of disease, so that eventually the bottom (or base) of the pocket reaches the CEJ. The pocket epithelium may be thin, even containing minute ulcers, so it is not surprising that *bleeding* may occur from these sites, often when a toothbrush or fibrous food touches the gum. Such bleeding is often slight, and may not worry the patient, but it is a principal indicator of disease and is never normal.

The low-grade type of gingival inflammation we have been describing is called *chronic gingivitis*. Most mouths probably have at least one site which shows some evidence of chronic gingivitis, usually where plaque removal is regularly inadequate or hampered in some way. It is common in children,

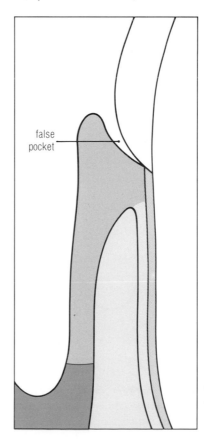

false pocket

Fig. 9.6 Appearance of gingiva in false pocket formation. Compare with Fig. 9.1.

often where teeth are erupting. In adults it also commonly occurs at the following sites:

- Lingually to lower molars (toothbrush access is limited by the tongue, and occasionally by a retching tendency) and incisors
- Buccally to upper molars (access limited by the ramus of the mandible and inside of the cheek)
- Where teeth are crowded or displaced
- Where poorly contoured fillings encroach on the gum margin
- Adjacent to orthodontic appliances
- Adjacent to partial dentures
- Where calculus has formed
- Where food particles commonly collect

A few patients always seem to have some gingival margin plaque and chronic gingivitis. In some patients, the gingival margins and papillae may eventually become firmer and paler, although remaining swollen, rounded, or blunted; if the amount of swelling increases the condition may be called 'chronic hyperplastic gingivitis', and the papillae are usually most noticeably affected (*Fig. 9.7*). Pregnancy, certain drugs, and various disorders (page 104), may promote the development of chronic gingival enlargement in some patients by exaggerating the usual response to plaque.

Again, the papillae are often most noticeably affected. Any degree of gingival enlargement of

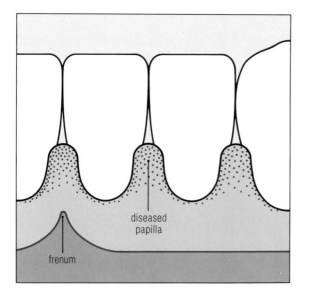

Fig. 9.7 Hyperplastic gingiva. (An isolated gingival swelling is often called an epulis).

course increases the depth of the pockets characteristic of chronic gingivitis, and sometimes may be severe enough to obscure the crowns of the teeth partially. Occasionally, an isolated swelling called an epulis (plural: epulides) may arise on the gum, perhaps as a localised response to plaque.

This section has been mainly concerned with the development and features of chronic gingivitis. Its treatment will be described on page 108. Types of acute gingivitis are described on page 101–103.

PERIODONTITIS

Periodontitis means inflammation of the periodontium.

With very few exceptions, the most important feature is that the disease process giving rise to periodontitis causes progressive and usually irreversible destruction of the bone supporting the teeth, loss of periodontal membrane and changes in the cementum.

Like chronic gingivitis, periodontitis in many individuals is a low-grade but insidious process causing few symptoms to alarm the patient until it is well advanced. However, a tooth affected by it may eventually lose so much bone that it becomes loose and may be lost.

At many sites, periodontitis appears to develop from gingivitis. Thus one reason for trying to treat gingivitis is to reduce the likelihood of periodontitis developing. Whereas gingivitis is reversible with appropriate treatment, periodontitis is irreversible — any portion of the supporting structures once lost cannot be predictably regained.

Although patterns vary, it is easiest first of all to describe chronic periodontitis as an extension of the disease process described for chronic gingivitis (page 95). When the base of the (false) pocket, characteristic of gingivitis, reaches the CEJ, bacteria there continue to produce substances which diffuse further and provoke superficial destruction of the bone margin. (This type of bony destruction is called 'resorption' and the bone is said to be 'resorbing'). As adjacent periodontal membrane also breaks down, junctional epithelium grows onto the cementum. This is followed in turn by an apical movement onto the root of the pocket base, the pocket of course being lined (as in gingivitis) by pocket epithelium. A pocket with its base on the root is called a *true pocket* (*Fig. 9.8*), and is characteristic of periodontitis. Note that a true pocket can only form after some bone has been resorbed, and the finding of a pocket extending beyond (apical to) the CEJ (to any distance) denotes the presence of periodontitis.

These changes tend to occur first of all in the bone between the teeth, particularly of the first permanent molar. A radiograph (X-ray film) might show a slight deterioration in the density of the crestal bone.

Clearly, at this stage of 'early' (or 'marginal') periodontitis, the involved tooth is still well supported by its remaining periodontium. If mobility were tested, one would expect it to be normal.

However, if left untreated (or inadequately treated), periodontitis will progress along the root, by an extension of the process already described, through stages which may be called 'moderate periodontitis' and then 'advanced periodontitis' until the remaining bone is insufficient to support the tooth any longer. In general, molar teeth tend to show a greater predisposition to periodontitis than non-molars because of the greater difficulty in cleaning them.

The patient's first indication of advancing periodontitis is often that the affected teeth start to move, tilt, or become loose. Adjacent affected teeth may become crowded, or drift apart causing spaces. They may extrude, meaning that they seem to grow out of their sockets. These features may increase where contact with opposing teeth is unfavourable.

During this entire process bone resorption may occur evenly at a site, creating a horizontal plane of residual bone (*Fig. 9.8*); this is called 'horizontal bone loss' and often affects adjacent teeth to an equal extent. The base (bottom) of the associated true pocket in such instances remains 'above' (coronal to) the resorbing bone, and is hence also called a 'supra-bony pocket'. Or sometimes the resorption may occur unevenly, creating a bony defect which slopes inwardly from its margin 'down' (apically) towards the root (*Figs. 9.9 and 9.10*); this is called 'vertical bone loss'. As may be expected, this irregular type of bone loss affects adjacent teeth (and even different parts of the same tooth) unequally. The base of the associated true pocket in such instances is at a more apical level than its bony margin, and is hence also called an 'infra-bony' (or 'intra-bony') pocket.

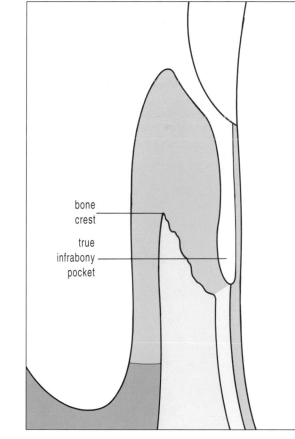

Fig. 9.9 *True infrabony pocket, showing the sloping level of the residual bone and the position of the base of the pocket relative to the bone crest. Compare with Figs. 9.1, 9.8, & 9.10.*

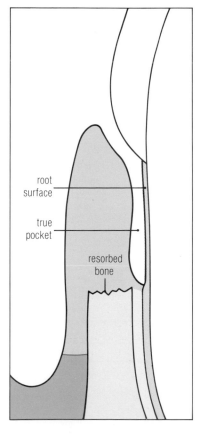

Fig. 9.8 *True pocket, with root surface involved and resorbed bone. (Note the 'horizontal' pattern of resorbed bone, and compare it with Figs. 9.1 and 9.9.) The pocket shown here, with its base 'above' the bone, is 'supra-bony'.*

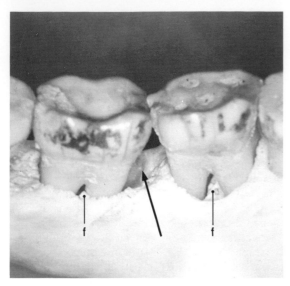

Fig. 9.10 *'Vertical' bone loss of the mesial root of a permanent mandibular molar (arrowed). The furcations of both molars (f) also show some bone loss.*

Variations in periodontitis

Any description of periodontitis is complicated by the fact that its presentation and behaviour vary widely in the population.

Five basic types of periodontitis have been described as in *Fig. 9.11*. We will say something about each type.

Pre-pubertal periodontitis (PP)

Unlike gingivitis, periodontitis is uncommon in healthy children. PP is rare. Teeth may be lost rapidly and in multiple.

Juvenile periodontitis (JP)

This uncommon disorder first manifests in teenagers, and usually has the following main features:

- Usually localised to first permanent molars and incisors, but may later involve other teeth
- Gingiva often appear healthy, but deep true pockets occur at above sites which bleed briskly on probing
- Radiographs of involved sites show deep vertical bone loss (infra-bony type; Fig. 9.10); patterns of bone loss are often similar on opposite sides of the same jaw
- Affected teeth may become mobile or drift
- Oral hygiene is often good
- Sparse subgingival plaque present, dominated by particular Gram-negative capnophilic rod-like organism which has high potential to cause periodontal destruction
- Females may be affected more than males
- Patients may have familial or ethnic predisposition, but have no known general disease
- Possibly inadequate response by white cells
- Prognosis may be poor where teeth are grossly involved or if treatment (page 107) is inadequate.

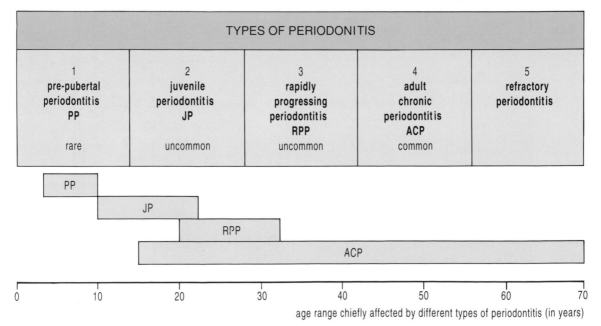

Fig. 9.11 Five basic types of periodontitis which have been described.

Rapidly progressive periodontitis (RPP)

This disorder, which is also rather uncommon, has the following main features:

- Gingiva often red, but oral hygiene is usually meticulous
- Multiple, deep, true pockets form rapidly
- Many teeth may be involved, which become mobile
- Brisk bleeding on probing and exudation of pus
- May be prone to periodontal abscesses (page 102)
- Radiographs show severe widespread bone loss of 'vertical' or 'horizontal' type
- Age of onset is uncertain, but the disorder often presents between 20 and 40 years of age, mainly affecting females
- No known general disease presents
- Disorder may cover a spectrum of similar diseases
- Various Gram-negative bacteria usually dominate subgingival plaque
- Prognosis is usually poor, with high susceptibility to recurrence in some individuals despite treatment (page 107).

Adult chronic periodontitis (ACP)

This is the commonest type of periodontitis. The earliest subtle evidence of disease occurs in the mid-teenage years, mesial to the first permanent molars. Thereafter it seems to progress through phases of varying activity (although this spasmodic pattern may not be so evident in retrospect), with some sites tending to become more extensively and persistently involved than others. Eventually, and usually by middle age, some teeth may require removal. This trend towards at least partial tooth loss may be arrested or retarded by appropriate treatment (pages 107–117), possibly preserving sufficient teeth to maintain adequate function and a good facial appearance without recourse to dentures.

The above disorders, apart from PP, are not always as distinct clinically as might be supposed, and what category a particular patient fits into is sometimes uncertain. It seems possible that RPP and ACP might together cover a range of 'periodontal diseases', which are different in some details but similar in others. However, the overall treatment plan (page 107) is largely the same.

Refractory periodontitis

This term is usually applied to a form of periodontitis which fails to respond to conventional treatment (page 117).

Susceptibility to periodontitis

You may be wondering if there is an explanation for the variations in periodontitis just described.

Generally, bone loss in periodontitis occurs in phases; periods of progression and stability alternate. Even in the same mouth, some sites may be deteriorating whilst others are stable. However, in retrospect, this spasmodic pattern may not be so evident. Also, it is hard to predict at present when any site may start to deteriorate.

This varying pattern, and the different degrees and types of disease, may be explained by alterations in the balance between the patient's resistance and the activity of different plaque microbes (*Fig. 9.12*).

The balance at a site may be tilted in favour of disease by:

1. Changes in the bacterial population

As mentioned earlier, even the tooth surface inside a false pocket in gingivitis harbours many different bacteria. These in time may create an altered environment which favours the multiplication of further types of bacteria able to initiate the changes associated with periodontitis. As, subsequently, true pockets

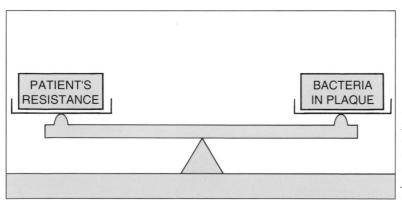

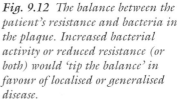

Fig. 9.12 The balance between the patient's resistance and bacteria in the plaque. Increased bacterial activity or reduced resistance (or both) would 'tip the balance' in favour of localised or generalised disease.

develop and deepen, bacterial films collect on the involved root surface (*Fig. 9.8*). At times this deep level plaque becomes dominated by bacteria with a high potential to cause damage, and consequently a phase of disease activity ensues, ceasing once balance is restored. Various Gram-negative anaerobic rod-like microbes and others, some showing movement, seem particularly involved in disease activity.

2. The patient's resistance may be impaired
Perhaps because of other illness, smoking, certain drugs, and possibly stress.

3. The patient may have an inherited limitation to cope with certain microbes

4. Certain products of a patient's defence mechanisms may inadvertently promote damage

The tendency towards disease will obviously increase if lowered resistance and increased microbial activity are combined. Balance may be restored if the patient's resistance improves or the bacterial changes stabilise. Treatment of course is directed at restoring the balance.

Clearly a younger patient with minimal plaque and advanced loss of alveolar bone is more suscepti-

ble to periodontitis than the older person whose teeth have good bony support despite extensive deposits of plaque and calculus. The more susceptible patient may also be more prone to disease recurrence or resistant to conventional treatment (refractory).

Gingival features in periodontitis
So far in this section on periodontitis we have said little about the appearance of the gingiva. This is because the gingival tissues often give no real indication of the extent of periodontitis which they conceal, and may have a variety of appearances, even at different sites in the same mouth. Thus the gingival margins and papillae may be swollen and either shiny and red or firm and pale. (The term 'combined pocket' is sometimes used where gingival enlargement and a true pocket occur together.) At other sites affected by periodontitis the gingival margin may recede, exposing part of the root (*Fig. 9.13*). Because of this recession, some patients say they are getting 'long in the tooth'.

Elsewhere the gingiva may regain, or retain, a semblance of health. Indeed, in some patients, there may be no clear evidence that their periodontitis was preceded by gingivitis.

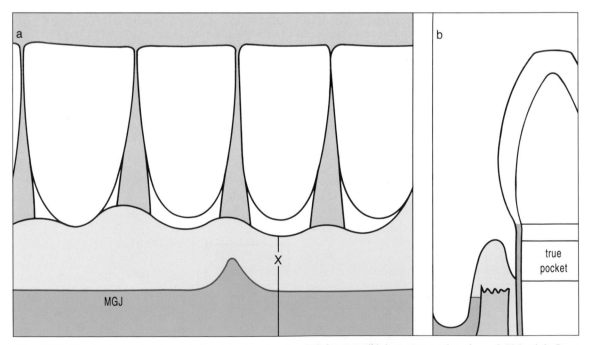

Fig. 9.13 *Gingival recession in periodontitis, exposing part of the root; (b) is a cross-section through X in (a). Some true pocketing remains. Compare with Figs. 9.5 and 9.8.*

Whatever the gingival appearance overlying periodontal destruction, blood may ooze from the pocket wall (as in gingivitis) and pus may form. These substances, as well as plaque products, calculus, and decomposing food particles in the pocket may give the patient an unpleasant taste and possible 'bad breath' (halitosis). Contact from the toothbrush or certain foods may stimulate obvious bleeding. Occasionally blood appears spontaneously. Some patients complain that they can 'suck' blood from their gums and others that it stains their pillows. Presumably some exudate is swallowed.

Clearly many signs and symptoms may accompany periodontitis. Some or all of the following may occur, even in the same patient:

- Bleeding (on toothbrushing, eating, or spontaneously)
- Pus formation
- Unpleasant taste and breath
- Discomfort (soreness, itching, dull ache)
- Colour changes of overlying gingiva (diagnostically unreliable)
- Gingival enlargement
- Gingival recession
- Looseness (mobility) and drifting of teeth
- Food packing or wedging between teeth
- Acute changes (ANUG and abscesses; see below)

Some patients still use the old word 'pyorrhoea' when teeth are getting loose, with pus formation and bleeding.

ACUTE DISORDERS OF THE PERIODONTIUM

Primary herpetic stomatitis
This infection, caused by the herpes simplex virus, sometimes presents as an acute infection of the mouth (stomatitis) which may involve the gingiva. It is commonest in infants and young adults.

When first infecting the body, the virus may provoke a severe inflammatory reaction which in the mouth presents with blisters on most soft tissues which soon ulcerate. If involved, the gingiva become red, swollen, and soft.

During the fortnight that this unpleasant disease lasts, the patient may be unwell, with raised temperature and enlarged lymph glands. The mouth may be sore enough to prevent eating. Healing thereafter appears total, but the virus remains dormant in the nerve, only to be reactivated at times by agents such as a head cold or sunlight. The familiar 'cold sore' on the lip is a typical result of this reactivation. The virus can be transmitted from a 'cold sore' to other individuals by contact, causing the primary infection just described in someone who has no immunity from previous contact. Susceptible dental personnel may develop on their fingers another unpleasant variant of the primary infection, the herpetic whitlow, if they touch a 'cold sore' on a patient. This is another good reason for wearing rubber gloves when treating patients (see also pages 11, 121, *Fig. 10.5*).

Pericoronitis
This means inflammation of the gingiva surrounding the crown of a tooth, usually during eruption. Plaque retention, food impaction, and direct damage are common causes. Pericoronitis may affect any tooth, but it is usually mild and resolves as the tooth erupts further. ('Teething', however, is often associated with herpetic stomatitis, page 119.)

However, the classic form of pericoronitis usually involves an emerging lower third molar tooth (wisdom tooth) which often fails to erupt fully and remains partly covered by a flap of gum. As a result:

- Plaque and food particles accumulate under the flap
- The affected gum becomes inflamed, swollen, and painful
- The upper wisdom tooth may bite onto the swollen tissues (Fig. 9.14)
- Resolution by natural means or by tooth cleaning is impossible

Without prompt and effective treatment (which may include irrigation under the flap, and removal of the opposing tooth, see page 140), pericoronitis involving the third molar may sometimes intensify, becoming complicated by ANUG, or by pus formation and serious spreading infection. In addition to severe pain, patients with pericoronitis sometimes have difficulty in opening the mouth (trismus).

Acute necrotising (ulcerative) gingivitis
This disorder, abbreviated to ANUG, has also been called Vincent's disease, AUG, ANG, 'trench mouth' (it afflicted soldiers engaged in trench warfare) and acute fusospirochaetal gingivitis (due to the main bacteria involved)!

It is the commonest acute disorder of the gum, causing rapid destruction (necrosis) and ulceration of the gingival papillae and sometimes the adjacent

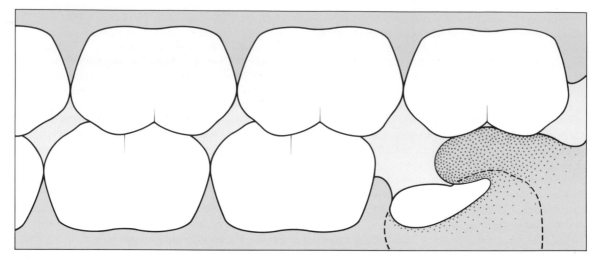

Fig. 9.14 *Pericoronitis affecting a partially erupted lower third molar. The gingival flap is constantly bitten on by the upper third molar.*

gingival margins (*Fig. 9.15*). It may be extensive, or limited to single sites, and may be associated with pericoronitis (page 102). On rare occasions it may destroy enough gum to expose bone, and may even spread into the cheek.

It mainly affects young adults. Common symptoms are:

- Bleeding (sometimes spontaneously) from involved sites
- Pain or soreness (sometimes severe)
- Characteristic unpleasant taste and odour
- Occasional raised temperature and malaise

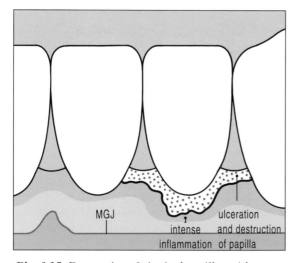

Fig. 9.15 *Destruction of gingival papillae with ulceration and spots of spontaneous haemorrhage, characteristic of ANUG.*

Poor oral hygiene is often a feature of ANUG. This may be the result, not the cause, of the disease. Nevertheless it is rare in clean mouths (and in such circumstances may denote serious systemic disease, page 108).

Other factors commonly predisposing to ANUG are:

- Chronic gingivitis or periodontitis
- Tobacco smoking
- Stress
- Acute viral disorders
- Reduced immunity
- Inadequate diet

In ANUG, predominating bacteria include spirochaetes (motile, spiral-shaped bacteria) and various Gram-negative microbes.

Even with treatment (page 108) ANUG is prone to recur.

Acute lateral periodontal abscess

This painful, localised, collection of pus develops at the side of the tooth (hence the term 'lateral') in the soft tissue wall of a true pocket. Thus they occur in sites already affected by chronic periodontitis. The patient complains of a swelling in the gum, often of rapid onset, and often accompanied by pain. The swelling is often red, but sometimes yellowish in the centre ('pointing') if about to burst and release pus. Occasionally the abscess drains spontaneously *via* the pocket entrance. Possible causes are:

- Change in composition of subgingival plaque
- Subgingival calculus preventing drainage (page 104)
- Damage to pocket wall (eg by pressure, scaling)

A tooth with this sort of abscess is usually vital and is not tender to bite on, unlike one with a *periapical* abscess caused by pulpal disease. However, treatment (page 108) is usually preceded by vitality testing, because periapical abscesses can occasionally point laterally or drain through the gum margin. Also as mentioned earlier, deep periodontal disease may occasionally involve the apex of the tooth.

FACTORS INFLUENCING THE ONSET, EFFECT, OR CONTROL OF DISEASE

Adequate plaque control is necessary for effective periodontal treatment. This is easier said than done. As already noted, some patients are particularly susceptible to disease, apparently being very reactive to even small amounts of subgingival plaque. Also certain factors localised to the mouth, or more generalised systemic factors, may either:

(a) alter the response of the tissues to the effects of plaque, or
(b) interfere with the removal of plaque

As the relevance of these factors needs to be considered when planning treatment, we will look at them now.

Local factors
- Limited mouth opening (small mouth, or because or trismus, pain, injury, or palsy)
- Gingival soreness or pain; sore mouth
- Access to gum margin restricted by narrow width of gum, inadequate space between lips, cheeks, or tongue, prominent frenum, or by retching when toothbrushing
- Type and position of teeth. Patients find access to molars difficult, and cleaning between them is difficult because they have broad contact areas
- Teeth which are crowded, tilted, rotated, or over-erupted
- Pre-existing reduction in bony support (dehiscences)
- Direct damage, such as by a tooth biting into the gum margin of an opposing tooth
- Inadequate lip seal or mouth breathing
- Rough enamel surface
- Caries
- Calculus (see below)

- Restorations with poor margins involving the gingival tissues
- Orthodontic appliances
- Dentures covering the gingival margin
- Exposed roots (roughness; sensitivity)
- Deep pockets

Deep pockets create problems because plaque accumulates in the surface roughness and hollows of the roots, and in the furcations (where the roots separate) of molar teeth and upper first premolars (*Fig. 9.10*).

Dental calculus (Fig. 9.16)
Calculus ('tartar') may be *supragingival* (at and above the gum margin) or *subgingival* (below the gum margin, inside a pocket). It is basically plaque which hardens by absorbing certain minerals. These are mainly calcium, phosphorus, and magnesium in various crystal forms particularly hydroxyapatite. The minerals come from saliva (supragingival calculus)

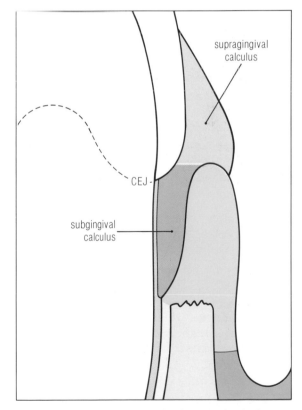

Fig. 9.16 Supragingival and subgingival calculus; a true pocket is present, filled with subgingival calculus.

and the exudate from the pocket wall (subgingival calculus).

Supragingival calculus may form extensively and quickly, particularly adjacent to the openings of salivary ducts; initially it tends to be rather soft and creamy in colour, but may later take up stains of dietary origin or from smoking. It is fairly easy to remove (page 112).

Subgingival calculus is usually stained black or greenish-red from blood products in the pocket. It forms slowly and is often hard to remove fully.

Calculus of either type is an important factor in the treatment of periodontal diseases because:

- Its surface is always covered with vital plaque
- Being rough, it promotes further plaque collection
- It retains bacteria close to the tissues where they do most harm
- It impairs drainage from the diseased sites
- It hinders access by saliva and oral hygiene devices

General factors

Any disorder which impairs the body's defence systems will either initiate or exacerbate disease. Examples are leukaemia, deficiencies of white cells, diabetes mellitus, hepatitis B, AIDS, and other disorders or drugs which directly or indirectly compromise the body's immune response.

The possibility of undiagnosed systemic disease is usually considered whenever periodontal disease exceeds what would be expected from the patient's age or amount of plaque present. Blood and urine investigations may therefore need to be arranged.

Hormonal changes in pregnancy may exaggerate the gingival response to plaque, causing a 'pregnancy epulis' (page 96) or more generalised papillary enlargement ('pregnancy gingivitis'). Drugs which may provoke gingival enlargement include phenytoin (to control epilepsy), nifedipine and diltiazem (to reduce high blood pressure), cyclosporin (page 59), and some oral contraceptives.

Patients with a history of rheumatic fever, endocarditis, heart murmur, valve replacement, and those

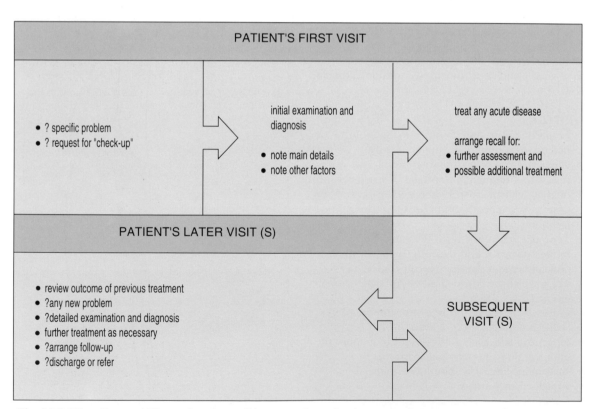

Fig. 9.17 'Flow diagram' illustrating the possible course of a patient's presentation, assessment, and treatment.

with organ transplants need antibiotic cover (page 108) for certain dental procedures.

Patients with natural or acquired blood clotting defects (eg haemophiliacs, those taking warfarin), and those with a history of radiotherapy of the head and neck, need special management.

Also, a patient's plaque removal may be hampered by physical handicaps (for instance deafness, blindness, absence of digits or limbs, spasticity, arthritis, neuromuscular disorders, stroke, and debilitating disease) and by certain mental handicaps which themselves may exacerbate periodontal disease (eg Down's syndrome).

DIAGNOSIS AND ASSESSMENT

A dentist's assessment of a patient's periodontal status is governed by whether the person is being seen for the first time or is keeping a recall appointment for treatment or follow-up. These stages are illustrated in *Fig. 9.17* as a 'flow diagram' (this general pattern may of course apply to other aspects of dentistry and to medical care in general).

At the first visit the dentist will note any symptoms reported by the patient (page 101), ask about any possible background factors (page 104), and carry out an extra-oral and intra-oral examination. Treatment may be prescribed at that stage (particularly for acute disorders) or arranged for a later date. At a later visit, the dentist will want to know what changes, if any, have occurred, especially if treatment had been given previously. A pattern of assessment as described earlier may again be necessary. Referral to a specialist may be indicated if the condition is severe or is deteriorating despite treatment.

Because gingival appearances are an unreliable indicator of the extent of any underlying periodontal destruction, dentists may probe between each tooth and its gingival margin for pockets (page 96), using a pocket measuring probe, of which many types are available.

Periodontal probing — initial assessment

The World Health Organization (WHO) probe is ball-ended, with a 2mm coloured band beginning 3.5mm from the tip (*Fig. 9.18*). As part of their initial assessment of a patient, some dentists use this probe for a 'Basic Periodontal Examination' — still sometimes called the Community Periodontal Index of Treatment Needs (CPITN). They divide the mouth into sixths (sextants) and the greatest severity of disease in each sextant is recorded numerically on a special six-boxed chart (*Fig. 9.19*). The dentist plans further treatment according to disease severity.

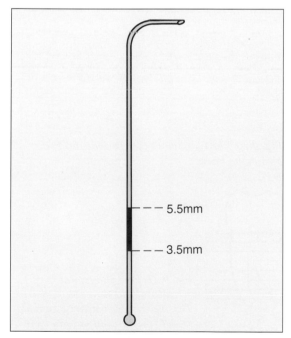

Fig. 9.18 The World Health Organization Periodontal Probe. The diameter of the ball at its tip is 0.5mm. If the entire band remains visible when the probe is inserted fully into a pocket, a score of 1 is recorded, or 2 if calculus is present. Score 3 is given if only part of the band remains visible, and 4 if none of the band remains visible. Please see Fig. 9.19.

- - - 5.5mm

- - - 3.5mm

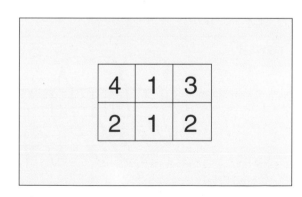

Fig. 9.19 Box chart for recording the highest value per sextant in a patient's mouth using the WHO probe (Fig. 9.18). In this example, the highest value in the upper right posterior sextant was 4, and in the upper left sextant was 3; both lower posterior sextants had top readings of 2, and the two anterior sextants were 1.

Periodontal probing — later assessment

Most pocket measuring probes are blunt-ended, calibrated, instruments of round or rectangular cross-section, and 10mm to 20mm in length. The Williams (14W) probe is shown in *Fig. 9.20*. Other measuring probes are 'pressure-sensitive', regulating the force which can be applied to probing. Electronic probes are also available which can produce a reading on a screen. Whatever method is used, the dentist will try to assess the distance between the CEJ and the pocket base (making appropriate allowance for the position of the gingival margin), thereby determining the 'loss of attachment' at that site; if this procedure is repeated at four or six points round a tooth it may be possible to assess what proportion of its root remains supported and thereby to estimate the prognosis. Readings may be transferred onto a special record chart (*Fig 9.21*), with which comparisons may be made later, during and after treatment.

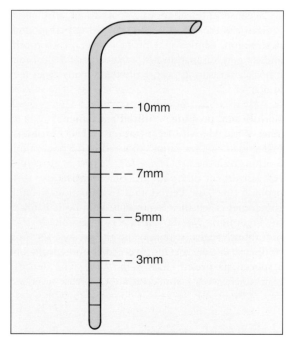

Fig. 9.20 *The Williams (14W) Periodontal Pocket Measuring Probe.*

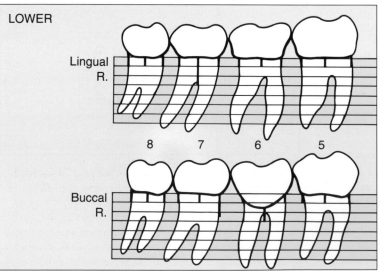
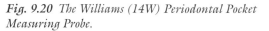

Fig. 9.21 *Part of a typical periodontal pocket recording chart. The lines are 2mm apart. Lingual to $\overline{876}|$ the gingival margin has a normal contour, and pockets are all 2mm deep, except for a 6mm pocket at the lingual mid-point of $\overline{7}|$. 3mm of recession and a 3mm pocket are recorded at the buccal mid-point of $\overline{6}|$; mesio-buccal to $\overline{7}|$ a 5mm pocket is shown. No other sites exceed 1mm.*

In a patient with periodontitis, bleeding from the gum margin on probing may denote inadequate oral hygiene, whereas bleeding from the base of the pocket denotes active disease (and, by inference, the presence of plaque at that level). Pus production means much the same.

Detailed assessments, which of course may not be necessary for every patient, may also include X-ray films (radiographs). Also special charts can be compiled which record pocket (probing) depths, sites which bleed (spontaneously or on probing), gingival recession, and tooth mobility. These details may be stored on computer, and comparisons made with them later, during and after treatment. The DSA who understands the significance of these readings from an appreciation of the diseases involved can give considerable help to the dentist.

Radiographs

Radiographs (X-ray films, roentgenograms) provide further information on the amount of bone destroyed or retained. The CEJ is a key landmark. As the distance between the healthy interdental bone crest and the CEJ rarely exceeds 2mm, any value exceeding this usually denotes periodontitis. However, bony variations which are buccal or lingual to the roots (such as dehiscences; see page 92) are rarely apparent. The gingival margin and pocket depths are not evident on radiographs which show only hard tissue detail. If we wish to know whether disease is progressing, we need comparable films taken at long intervals; this information cannot be obtained on one occasion (although susceptibility may be estimated; see page 100). Within these limitations, radiographs generally show the following:

- Variations in the density of bony margins
- Horizontal and vertical bone loss
- Bone loss between the roots of a molar tooth
- Calculus on the roots
- Approximal caries, on crowns or roots
- Ledges on fillings
- Combined periapical and periodontal changes
- Unerupted teeth
- Unknown disease (for example, cysts)

Mobility or drifting of teeth

Additional assessment and management may be needed if teeth are drifting or becoming loose. Possible causes are:

(a) Normal bone, but the patient has a habit of grinding or clenching the teeth

(b) Reduced bone levels as a result of:
- dehiscences and/or
- periodontitis
(c) As in (b), but the patient also grinds or clenches the teeth
(d) Other diseases affecting tooth support (eg cysts)

Other investigations

Because pulpal changes may sometimes present as a periodontal problem or a tooth may become non-vital as a consequence of advanced periodontitis, a dentist may test the vitality of any tooth where periodontal pockets appear to involve the root apex. Combined endodontic and periodontal therapy may be needed.

Some dentists collect samples of plaque, using it to instruct and motivate patients, as well as a further aid to diagnosis. Also, as mentioned earlier, techniques are available for analysing gingival fluid, which may give information on bacterial products and defence substances as well as identifying other 'markers' of disease activity and potential.

OUTLINE OF TREATMENT STAGES

Note any relevant medical history

Control any acute disease

Control chronic disease by:
- Effective plaque control by patient
- Removal of calculus and subgingival plaque
- Attend to modifying factors
- Periodontal surgery
    Gingivectomy
    Flaps
    Grafts and frenectomy
- Other procedures

Refractory periodontitis

Maintenance and follow-up care

PERIODONTAL TREATMENT

The patient's medical status

The dentist will usually review a patient's medical history (including drugs) regularly (see Chapter 4 and page 104).

The same, stringent, cross-infection controls in the surgery (page 11) should nowadays be applied to all patients. However, additional safeguards may be needed for some immunocompromised patients.

Certain patients (pages 54 and 105) need *antibiotic cover* for scaling, root planing, surgery, endodontics, and tooth removal. Suitable prophylaxis is usually provided by amoxycillin oral powder (3g) made up into a drink or by clindamycin capsules (600mg); these preparations are taken one hour before the procedure begins. Sometimes alternative preparations are needed.

Control of acute disease

Patients with pain, swelling, and other features of acute disease require prompt treatment.

Acute herpetic stomatitis requires anti-viral medication and possibly soothing mouthwashes. Clinically it resolves completely (but see page 101).

Pericoronitis may be controlled by irrigating under the inflamed flap with antiseptic liquids. An opposing tooth which is traumatising the flap may be removed initially or later, or its cusps may be reduced as a preliminary measure. If infection is more severe, antimicrobial drugs (see below) may be required. In due course the partly erupted tooth may require removal. During these stages, the DSA should be aware of what appropriate instruments may need laying up.

ANUG and acute lateral periodontal abscesses (and sometimes pericoronitis) usually develop in tissue which is already chronically inflamed. However, patients often do not realise this and assume that the entire disease has been eradicated once the acute phase has subsided. In fact, the tissues have merely reverted to a chronically inflamed, symptomless, state in which, without additional therapy, acute changes may again develop.

Persuading patients to realise the true situation may require counselling by dental personnel in which a DSA should be able to play an important part.

Nowadays, the initial treatment for severe ANUG is usually with antimicrobial drugs (as with pericoronitis), such as penicillin (unless the patient is allergic to it), erythromycin, or metronidazole. Penicillin is often given as amoxycillin, and the usual dosage of this is a 250mg capsule three times daily for five days. Metronidazole is often more effective than the other drugs, and its usual dosage is a 200mg tablet three times daily for five days. Patients should not take alcohol during treatment with metronidazole. This drug is not normally given to pregnant patients. Tetracyclines are unsuitable for treating these acute disorders.

In the case of ANUG, initial treatment may also include careful and gentle cleansing of the involved teeth, using an ultrasonic scaler (page 112), but the gingiva may be too sore to tolerate this. An antiseptic mouthwash, particularly sodium perborate powder (Bocasan®) dissolved in water, may help to reduce the acute phase.

An inadequate response to treatment, or rapid recurrence, may denote a serious underlying disease (such as diabetes, leukaemia, or AIDS).

The dentist will almost certainly decide to test the vitality of a tooth (page 69) with an acute lateral periodontal abscess, and the DSA should have the appropriate instruments ready. A radiograph may also be needed. The abscess may also need opening and draining, for which topical or local anaesthesia may be needed as well as scalpel, swab, and suction. Unless the tooth is to be removed shortly, antimicrobial therapy (usually metronidazole, as before) may be needed in addition to other follow-up measures (page 113).

Recurrent or multiple abscesses may also necessitate tests for underlying disease.

Control of chronic disease
Effective plaque control by the patient

Many patients believe that tooth loss is inevitable with 'gum disease', a prospect that few face with equanimity, although the main fear is usually an alteration of appearance rather than loss of eating ability. With adequate treatment the progress of periodontitis can usually be slowed down or even halted, and such reassurance may encourage patients to help themselves by effective removal of supragingival plaque if present.

Patients' attitudes towards plaque control (and dental care in general) are often complex, influenced by family and social background and other factors such as time and financial priorities.

Nevertheless patients need to understand about plaque, particularly regarding its effect in their own mouths. Advice given to one patient may not be appropriate for another, as amounts of plaque and levels of disease vary. The DSA can help by tactfully reinforcing advice given by the dentist and hygienist.

Removing supragingival plaque is the patient's responsibility, so they need advice on appropriate tooth cleaning aids and methods of use (*Fig. 9.22*) Conventional toothbrushes should be small enough to give comfortable access to all gingival margins; these sites, and in the embrasures, are often missed by faulty brushing (*Fig. 9.23*). Sensitivity and other factors (page 96) may limit brushing. A popular method of brushing was devised by C C Bass and is known by his name (*Fig. 9.24*): the brush is held at about 45° to the long axis of the tooth, with most of the filaments resting on the tooth close to the gum margin. Gentle pressure causes some filaments to enter the pocket opening. With the light pressure maintained, the brush head is activated with small rotatory or to-and-fro movements of the hand, dislodging plaque at and below the gum margin and in the embrasures. After counting up to five or more at one site, the brush may be swept towards the occlusal surface before moving to the next site. Other tooth brushing methods are just as valid if they remove all supragingival plaque without damaging the gum. Teeth should be brushed at least once a day (immediately before going to bed) and preferably also at another time (after breakfast); brushing more often than this is not essential. An orderly sequence of brushing round the mouth, whatever method is preferred, is better than random methods which often miss some sites. Brushing too vigorously, or incorrectly, may damage the gum and contribute to gingival recession (*Fig. 9.5*). Bending or enlarging toothbrush handles may be helpful, especially if patients have access problems.

Early plaque is invisible, but special tablets ('disclosing tablets') are available which, when chewed by patients, release a dye which highlights the plaque, and so makes its removal easier. The DSA may remind the patient that a smear of petroleum jelly on the lips will prevent them from becoming stained. Whether disclosants are used or not, patients should be encouraged to look into their mouths whilst brushing, by standing in front of a mirror and pulling the lips and cheeks out of the way with their free hand.

Patients also need encouragement to clean between their teeth in order to protect the vulnerable approximal area from plaque accumulation. This requires the use of floss, and the dentist or hygienist will usually advise on the type of floss and correct technique. Despite instruction, some patients find flossing difficult, in which case a floss-holder may prove useful.

Where spaces have formed approximally between the gum and contact area, single-tufted 'interspace' brushes, spiral-wound 'interdental' brushes (often nick-named 'bottle brushes'), wood sticks, thickened

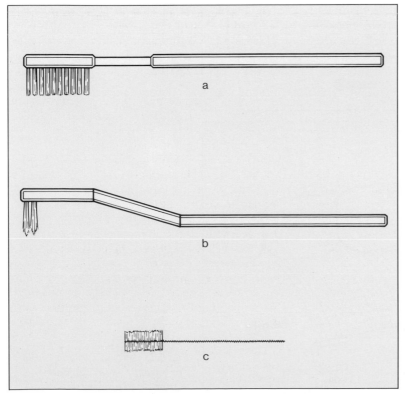

Fig. 9.22 *Three types of toothbrush: (a) conventional 'multi-tufted'; (b) interspace; (c) spiral-wound for interdental cleaning.*

floss, or tape may be useful. Spiral-wound brushes are good at cleaning hollows in the mesial and distal root surfaces, particularly of molar teeth.

Chlorhexidine mouthwash (0.2% solution) has proven antiplaque activity but it has a bitter taste, may make the soft tissues sore, and stains the teeth. The disadvantages may be minimised by using it less frequently, and restricting its application to needy sites, perhaps applying it on cotton buds. Other mouthwashes are available but, in general, have only minimal additional benefit to proper toothbrushing. None reliably enters subgingival sites.

Antiplaque toothpastes, some containing 'Triclosan', may be of some benefit in controlling supragingival deposits, but do not make proper toothbrushing unnecessary. Like other toothpastes (dentifrices) their effect subgingivally is probably only slight. Some other toothpastes are claimed to inhibit calculus formation.

Electric toothbrushes and pulsating irrigating devices may be useful to patients with limited dexterity.

Removal of supragingival plaque will normally promote complete resolution of chronic inflammation of the gingival margin, whether associated with false or true pockets, as gingiva has excellent powers of recuperation. If distortion of the gingival margin, produced by disease, does not resolve, attention to possible modifying factors (page 112) and surgery may be needed.

Removal of calculus and subgingival plaque

Whilst removal of soft supragingival deposits (plaque and food particles) is the responsibility of a properly-instructed able-bodied patient, removal of all calculus and subgingival plaque is the responsibility of the dentist or hygienist. Patients cannot remove plaque from inside pockets unless they are very shallow.

The DSA should be familiar with conventional scaling instruments. Examples are (*Fig. 9.25*):

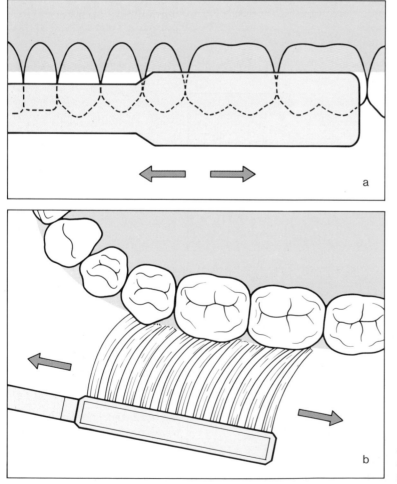

Fig. 9.23 *Incorrect toothbrushing leaves plaque at (a) the gum margin and (b) between the teeth.*

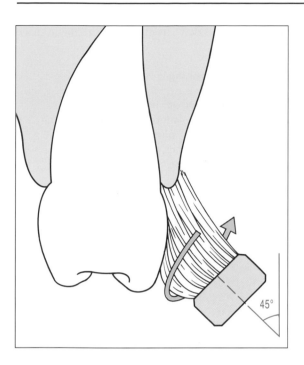

Fig. 9.24 The 'Bass' method of toothbrushing, the most suitable for controlling periodontal disease.

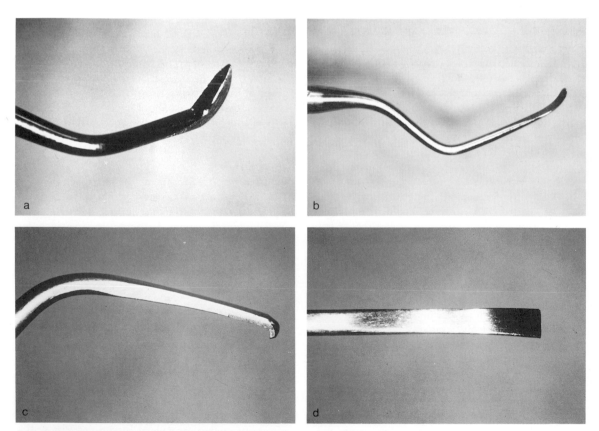

Fig. 9.25 Tips of four types of scaling instruments: (a) Jaquette; (b) Curette; (c) Hoe; (d) Push scaler.

- 'Push' (Spring or G1) scaler, with single cutting edge per blade, used between the lower incisors
- Dental hoe, with single cutting edge per blade, usually tipped with tungsten carbide to maintain sharpness
- Jaquette scaler, with a heavy triangular blade having two cutting edges
- Sickle scaler, a fine, elongated, curving instrument, pointed at the tip, and with two cutting edges
- Curette, with an elongated, slightly curved, spoon-like blade, having one or two cutting edges

The calculus probe, which has a fine shank with a sharp curve at the end, is sometimes mistaken for a scaling instrument!

This list is not exhaustive; various instruments of similar design, but of different sizes (and names), are available. Instruments may be conveniently classified into two groups: for supragingival work (large, heavy, blades) and for subgingival work (fine, narrow, blades, some specially designed to reach to the base of deep pockets and into furcation areas). Unless they have tungsten carbide tips, scalers need sharpening regularly to be fully effective. This work may be entrusted to the DSA.

To remove large amounts of calculus quickly, some dentists use ultrasonic scalers. Rapid vibrations of the tip (25,000 per second) are produced by mechanisms which in one type incorporates electromagnetic material and in another a quartz crystal. The profuse water spray which cools both types helps to lift materials off the tooth surface and also irrigates the site. High volume aspiration is needed, and the DSA should wear protective spectacles and a face mask to protect against the potentially harmful aerosol. The patient's clothing should be protected by a waterproof cover. Ultrasonic scalers should not be used on patients with cardiac pacemakers. Other methods of cleaning tooth surfaces rapidly are available. During *any* scaling procedure, patients need adequate eye protection.

Scaling denotes the removal of hard or soft deposits *on* the tooth surface and is usually followed by polishing. However, root surfaces, seen microscopically, are rough and pitted; microbes in these pits may not be removed by scaling. Also certain of their products may impregnate the outer layer of the cementum. Therefore, in addition to scaling (and perhaps on a different occasion), dentists may plane such roots using fine scaling instruments such as curettes. *Root planing* is slow, meticulous, work, and

the patient is likely to need a local anaesthetic (page 127).

Scaling and polishing

> ### Lay-up (with patient's records)
> 1. Scalers: push, Jaquette, periodontal hoes, sickle, curettes, ultrasonic with tips
> 2. Cotton wool rolls and pellets
> 3. Disclosing tablets/solution
> 4. Toothbrush
> 5. Dental floss
> 6. Spiral-wound brushes/interspace brushes
> 7. Wooden interdental sticks
> 8. Periodontal pocket-measuring and calculus probes
> 9. Fluoride prophylactic paste
> 10. Right-angled slow or special handpiece
> 11. Polishing brush and cup, hand mirror
> 12. Saliva ejector, dental napkins

After use, all scalers need to be scrupulously cleaned to remove debris and blood. If handling these instruments, DSAs need to take great care to avoid puncturing their skin, such as by wearing heavy-duty protective gloves. After being cleaned, scalers need to be properly autoclaved.

The removal of microbial deposits from the tooth surface arrests the disease in most instances. As the gingival inflammation resolves during healing, bleeding becomes less. Shrinkage of the gum margin also occurs; this may expose root surfaces which could be sensitive (*Figs. 9.13 and 9.31*).

Other factors

We have already mentioned that other factors (page 103) may impair scaling and healing. As far as possible dentists will try to reduce 'plaque retentive' areas by the gingival margins. Such measures may include:

- Smoothing rough enamel
- Treating carious cavities
- Reducing or replacing rough or excessive margins on restorations
- Modifying any bridges, orthodontic appliances, or partial dentures, if possible, where they are enhancing plaque accumulation.

It may not be possible to alter many of the factors listed on page 104, and the patient needs to understand therefore that the outcome of treatment may be limited. This, of course, may be particularly true of various medical or general conditions, although a dentist and doctor may liaise where necessary; for example gingival enlargement related to certain drugs for high blood pressure or epilepsy may decrease with alternative medication. 'Pregnancy gingivitis' (page 96) usually resolves completely after childbirth, provided that any plaque and calculus is removed.

Some dental factors involved in periodontal diseases may require more extensive measures (page 117).

Periodontal surgery

For various reasons, the measures already described (basically improvements in oral hygiene, and supragingival and subgingival removal of calculus and plaque) may not be entirely successful. This is more likely when:

- Gingival contour has become distorted
- More active or advanced disease is present (including Juvenile Periodontitis and Rapidly Progressive Periodontitis)
- Pockets are deep or irregular
- Pockets involve furcations
- Access is restricted
- Time is insufficient
- Patients experience discomfort
- Choice of instruments is limited

In such circumstances various other measures may be helpful, including surgical procedures which will now be described.

• Gingivectomy

Gingivectomy means totally excising the gum forming the pocket wall, thus eliminating the pocket. After the site has been anaesthetised (page 128), puncture marks are made (with Crane-Kaplan forceps or a probe) indicating the level of the base of the pocket (*Fig. 9.26a*). A blade held obliquely is then drawn through the tissues to be resected, using successive puncture marks as a guide; the tip of the blade touches the tooth at the base of the pocket during this procedure (*Fig. 9.26b*). Some dentists place the blades in special Blake Knife handles or similar carriers. An electrosurgery electrode may be used instead of a blade for gingivectomy.

Although removing the site of disease, gingivectomy creates a large wound which initially may be painful, prone to bleed, slow to heal, and susceptible to infection. Gingivectomy wounds, therefore, need covering during healing with a periodontal dressing or pack.

False pockets and hyperplastic gingiva (distorting the gingival contour) may be treated by this

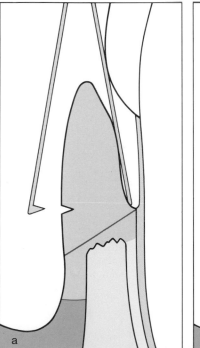
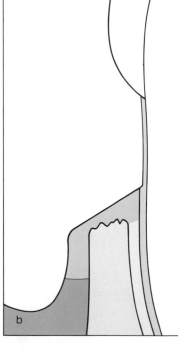

Fig. 9.26 Gingivectomy. (a) The base of the suprabony pocket has been indicated by a puncture mark made by the Crane-Kaplan forceps. The incision is shown by the red line. The blade meets the tooth at an angle of about 45°. (b) After gingivectomy, the root is left exposed.

method. However gingivectomy is less suitable for true pockets because roots become exposed (*Fig. 9.13*). Also, bone defects remain hidden. Excision of deep pockets may compromise the mucogingival junction (MGJ) (page 93).

• *Flaps*

Simple flaps conserve the gingiva whilst giving access to the base of the pocket, root surface and any furcations, and bone defects. After the site has been anaesthetised (page 128), the stages are as follows:

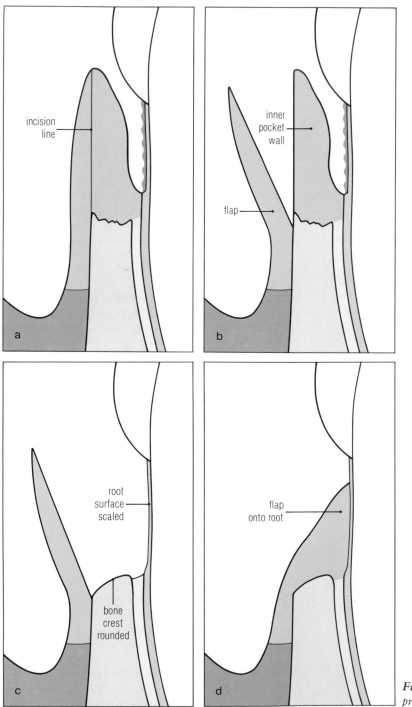

Fig. 9.27 Stages (a)–(d) of a flap procedure in cross-section.

1. A blade entering the gingival margin near to the pocket entrance passes almost vertically to the resorbed bone crest and, maintaining this position, is drawn through the tissues from one tooth to the next in the area being treated (*Fig. 9.27a*).
2. The 'outer wall' of the gum, thus freed from the 'inner (pocket) wall', is turned carefully aside as a flap, until the bone is visible (*Fig. 9.27b*).
3. The 'inner (pocket) wall' of soft tissue is removed (with blades or curettes). If a similar flap has been raised on the other side of the teeth in question, any residual soft tissue between their roots will also be removed.
4. The exposed root surfaces are thoroughly scaled and planed, using conventional and ultrasonic scalers (*Fig. 9.27c*).
5. Any bulky or sharp bone margins may be lightly rounded (using a large rosehead bur cooled by saline) to enhance better flap return (*Fig. 9.27c*).
6. The flap is placed back against the treated root surface, and sutured through each interdental space to gum on the other side (*Fig. 9.27d*).

Λ dressing is often not needed. In healing, such flaps may partially or completely reseal themselves to the clean root surface by a long junctional epithelium. To the extent that such flaps re-cover the roots, they help to avoid the problems mentioned earlier.

The flap just described has several variations. For example the blade may be directed more obliquely within the soft tissues to the bone margin, or it may be placed *in* the pocket (between root and pocket wall) to sever the soft tissue attachment at the base of the pocket. A flap may be mobilised further by being freed from the bone to a point beyond the MGJ (*Fig. 9.28a*); it can then be moved apically until its margin lies over the resorbed bone margin; this 'apically respositioned flap' conserves soft tissue but leaves roots exposed (*Figs. 9.28b and 9.13*). Flaps mobilised in this way may also be moved coronally or laterally, usually to cover roots partially exposed by previous gingival recession (*Fig. 9.5*, see also grafts, page 116).

Flaps may also provide access for putting bone chips in bone defects or placing special membranes over the bone margin and root to promote the formation of new bone and periodontal membrane by a process called 'Guided Tissue Regeneration' (*Fig. 9.29*). Some membranes need removing later, after their effect is complete, but others can be left.

Raising a flap may show, or confirm, that bone loss is so extensive that the tooth is better removed at that time.

Where bone loss particularly involves one root of a multirooted tooth, that root may be separated from the rest of the tooth via a flap procedure and

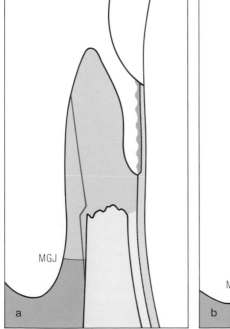
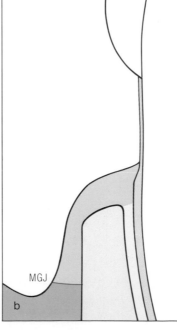

Fig. 9.28 Apically respositioned flap in cross-section. Note the new level of MGJ.

removed, usually after prior endodontic therapy of the other root(s).

Flaps may also include edentulous areas as part of a procedure to place implants (page 151).

• Other soft tissue surgery

Where there is minimal width of gum, such as at a site of gingival recession, a *gingival graft* may provide extra width and enhance plaque control (*Fig. 9.30*). The site to receive the graft is first prepared and then a thin piece of tissue of the right size is brought from another site, often the hard palate, and stabilised in its new position by sutures or special adhesive, usually covered by a dressing. Gingival grafts tend to remain pale compared with the adjacent tissues.

A prominent frenum may be better removed *(frenectomy)* if it is involved in a diastema or is preventing a toothbrush from reaching an area effec-

tively. Where gingival recession involves a frenum, frenectomy may be part of a gingival grafting procedure (see below).

Assisting at surgery

In all surgical procedures the DSA has an invaluable part to play in monitoring the patient, retracting tissues, providing effective aspiration, irrigating the operative site, and in the exchange of appropriate instruments.

For a simple flap procedure, instruments such as the following may be sufficient:

1. Aspirating local anaesthetic syringe and solution (*Fig. 12.1*).
2. Scalpel handle
3. Disposable blades
4. Periosteal elevator
5. Tissue forceps
6. Needle holder
7. Needle with silk or nylon suturing material
8. Surgical scissors
9. Scaling instruments

This list is not exhaustive, and other instruments may be added or substituted to suit the dentist's

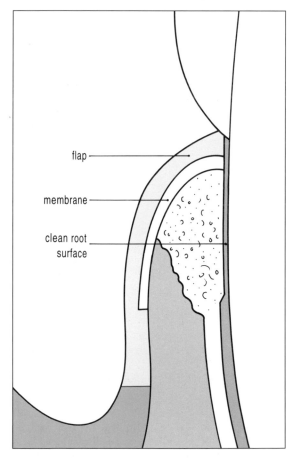

Fig. 9.29 *A special membrane placed as shown may promote formation of new bone, periodontal membrane, and cementum underneath (dotted area).*

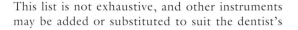
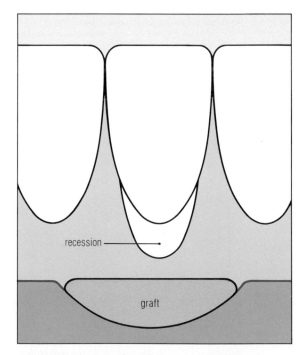

Fig. 9.30 *A gingival graft is often taken from the gingiva of the hard palate. It is used to widen the existing gingiva and to facilitate toothbrushing.*

preference. Special instruments and materials are needed for more advanced procedures.

The DSA should be familiar at a practical level with periodontal dressings and their mixing properties.

INSTRUCTIONS TO PATIENTS AFTER PERIODONTAL SURGERY

Until any numbness wears off, be careful not to damage the treated area, lip, inside of the cheek, or tongue.

Avoid eating on the treated area for at least **one week.**

For the rest of the FIRST day, avoid hot liquids and food.

Any discomfort should respond to paracetamol. It is better to avoid aspirin.

If bleeding occurs, apply gentle but firm pressure to the area for at least five minutes using gauze or a clean cotton handkerchief. Do not rinse.

The day after surgery, rinse gently round your mouth with warm saltwater every four to six hours, and similarly on subsequent days.

Do not brush the treated area for the first week. Instead, hold 10ml of 0.2% chlorhexidine mouthwash (Corsodyl®) in the area for one minute, at least once daily (at bedtime). Keep all your other teeth clean using your usual method.

If a periodontal dressing has been placed in the area, try to avoid dislodging it. However, if it becomes loose, remove it, and use chlorhexidine mouthwash as above.

At your next appointment after surgery, any stitches and dressings will be removed, and the area will be checked and cleaned. It is very important to keep this appointment. Occasionally a further dressing may be needed.

Maintaining a high standard of oral cleanliness and plaque removal is **essential** during the first week and thereafter to encourage and maintain good healing.

If any problems arise, or if you need advice, contact the surgery without delay.

Other procedures
Apart from surgery, or in addition to it, the following measures may occasionally be indicated:

- Orthodontic correction of malaligned teeth if their malposition is thought to be hindering adequate plaque control or is a result of periodontal disease.
- Grinding the occlusal surfaces of teeth which either have periodontal disease or which are at times in unfavourable contact with such teeth.
- Endodontic treatment either where pulp death is contributing to periodontal problems or where periodontal treatment may devitalise the tooth.
- Treating sensitive roots with special pastes, solutions or varnishes (several of which contain fluorine compounds) or with a laser. Some dentists cover sensitive roots with restorations *(Fig 9.31)*.
- Where two teeth share a deep pocket, removal of one tooth may preserve the other for a longer period.
- Provision of a gum shield may help to control hyperplasia associated with inadequate lip seal.
- Syringing chlorhexidine into deep pockets.
- Where periodontitis is particularly active (signs of severe inflammation, such as profuse and/or extensive bleeding from pockets on probing) or rapid, especially where plaque is not abundant, *antimicrobial therapy* may eradicate bacteria, some of which may have penetrated the pocket wall, overwhelmed the body's defence mechanisms, or taken advantage of a weakness in these mechanisms. A long course of tetracycline (or a derivative of it) may prove useful, and is particularly indicated for Juvenile Periodontitis or Rapidly Progressive Periodontitis because it is active against the bacteria involved. Other antimicrobials in use for active disease include a combination of amoxycillin and metronidazole for five days, or another preparation with amoxycillin. (Some antibiotics, notably tetracycline, may reduce the efficacy of oral contraceptives, and some patients may need to be warned about this.) Antimicrobial preparations which can be put directly into periodontal pockets are being developed.

Refractory periodontitis
This term has come into use in recent years to describe periodontitis which fails to respond to conventional therapy, progressing despite treatment.

As tissues exist in a state of balance between the host's resistance and microbial activity, any persistence of disease after removal of plaque may indicate the presence of resistant or inaccessible microbes, or diminished host resistance. Therefore various blood tests and urine analysis may be necessary as well as a review of treatment given. Antimicrobial therapy (described in the previous section) may be indicated.

Maintenance and follow-up care

No form of periodontal treatment, including surgery, prevents recurrence of disease. Patients need to be aware that, if plaque re-forms, signs of disease will re-appear. Such an eventuality may not mean therefore that previous treatment was insufficient or incorrect.

The frequency of recall visits depends on the susceptibility of patients to disease (page 100), their extent of motivation and dexterity, and other factors such as relevant medical conditions. Patients who are prone to periodontal diseases may need to be seen frequently.

Inevitably, some teeth may require extraction, even after intensive efforts to retain them have been made. However, loose teeth can often be retained for some considerable time, giving at least partial function, provided that the residual periodontium is healthy (after treatment), and that they are not becoming a nuisance or liability to the patient and the remaining dentition. Simple splints or retainers may provide support for some mobile teeth, and may prevent further movement, although they may hinder plaque removal.

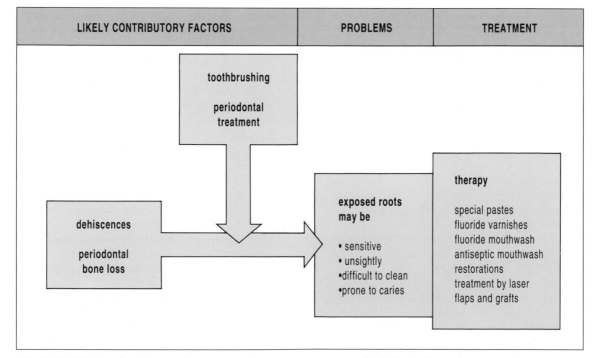

Fig. 9.31 *Likely cases, effects, and treatment of root exposure as a result of gingival recession.*

10. Diseases of the Oral Mucosa

MOUTH ULCERS

Mouth ulcers are usually the result of injury caused, for example, by biting. Recurrent aphthae are also common. Most mouth ulcers are painful but not of any consequence. However, it is important to ensure that they are not caused by drugs or serious diseases of blood, skin, or the intestines, infections or even tumours (*Fig. 10.1*).

Local causes of ulcers

Children may bite their lip while under a local dental anaesthetic; they should, therefore, be warned against this. Occasionally, dentures or orthodontic plates produce ulcers. In this case, they should be adjusted to help healing of the ulcer.

Any form of injury may produce ulcers. New dentures often produce ulcers in the sulcus; these dentures should be eased to help the ulcer to heal.

An ulcer that does not heal within three weeks should be biopsied by the dentist or a specialist, since it may be a tumour or another serious condition.

Recurrent aphthae

These affect about one person in four out of the entire population. They usually start in childhood or adolescence, persisting until the later 30s and sometimes for life. Most aphthae are small round ulcers that last approximately one week and occur in the cheek and lip mucosa, or under the tongue. As similar ulcers are sometimes caused by general disease, blood tests often need to be carried out.

Treatment

Chlorhexidine mouthwashes;
Corticosteroid pellets, paste, mouthwashes or sprays.

Cancer

Oral cancer is uncommon in Britain, but particularly common in India and other parts of Asia. It usually affects the lower lip or the tongue. The cause is unknown but several factors may be involved, summarised in *Fig. 10.2*.

As lip cancer is usually recognised and treated promptly, most patients can be cured. However, the cure rate is lower in tongue cancer. Oral cancer may appear as an ulcer, a lump, or as a red, white or brown patch. It spreads to the jaw and lymph nodes in the neck, where it may cause a tumour. Any ulcer lasting more than three weeks, as well as most lumps and white or coloured lesions, are biopsied by the dentist or specialist in order to exclude cancer.

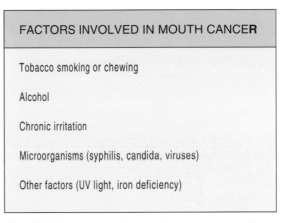

CAUSES OF MOUTH ULCERS

Local (e.g. denture trauma)

Recurrent aphthae

Cancer

Systemic disease (infections/blood/gastrointestinal/skin disease)

Drugs

Fig. 10.1 Mouth ulcers may be the result of several factors.

FACTORS INVOLVED IN MOUTH CANCER

Tobacco smoking or chewing

Alcohol

Chronic irritation

Microorganisms (syphilis, candida, viruses)

Other factors (UV light, iron deficiency)

Fig. 10.2 Summary of factors that may cause oral cancer.

Treatment

Radiotherapy, and/or surgery.

General diseases

There are rare, but important causes of mouth ulcers.

Infections

Children get mouth ulcers due to viral infections, particularly herpes simplex stomatitis. This is a common cause of teething. Patients develop ulcers, gingivitis and a high temperature, with a generalised feeling of illness. Antivirals may be useful, but the most important steps are to ensure sufficient liquid intake and to keep temperature under control (with

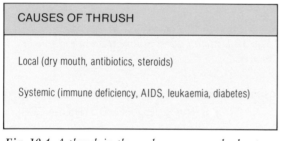

CAUSES OF WHITE PATCHES

Thrush	Leucoplakia
Lichen planus	Cancer

Fig. 10.3 *White patches of the mucous membrane may be due to local systemic factors or infections.*

CAUSES OF THRUSH

Local (dry mouth, antibiotics, steroids)

Systemic (immune deficiency, AIDS, leukaemia, diabetes)

Fig. 10.4 *A thrush in the oral mucosa may be due to local or systemic factors.*

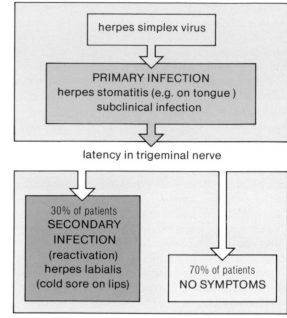

Fig. 10.5 *Herpes virus infection; this may be primary, secondary or asymptomatic.*

paracetamol since children should not use aspirin) so that the child does not get 'fever fits'. Saliva from infected patients can transmit the infection.

Other uncommon infections that may cause ulcers include rare serious diseases such as AIDS, syphilis and tuberculosis.

Blood disease
Anaemia and leukaemia may cause mouth ulcers.

Intestinal disease
Diseases of the small intestine (for example, coeliac disease) interfere with digestion and absorption of food, causing mouth ulcers.

Skin disease
Some skin diseases, particularly lichen planus, may affect the mouth and cause ulcers. Other skin disorders may be potentially harmful more generally; these are diagnosed by the dentist after history-taking, examination or biopsy, and urine/blood tests. They are treated by the dentist in cooperation with the doctor or specialist.

WHITE PATCHES
White patches in the mouth are usually caused by thickening of the mucosa. Their main importance is that some develop into cancer. Others are caused by fungal infection and may provide an early sign of immunological problems such as AIDS. Causes of white patches in the mouth are shown in *Fig. 10.3*.

Thrush
Thrush looks like milk curds, and the white patches can easily be wiped off the mucosa. The mouth is often sore.

Newborn babies may be infected by the fungus *Candida*, as they have not had time to develop immunity to it. In older patients, any changes causing dryness (for example, drugs and radiation), or interference with the bacterial flora (for example, antibiotics), may cause thrush (*Fig. 10.4*). The dentist should locate and treat the cause; antifungals may also be prescribed. In some patients, thrush may occur due to a more serious disease (for example, AIDS, leukaemia and diabetes).

Leucoplakia
This is the name given to white patches that cannot be wiped off the mucosa. They may be caused by irritation, smoking, or other unknown factors, Leucoplakia usually affects the cheek mucosa. It is benign usually, but about two to four in every hundred turn into cancer. The dentist should arrange a

biopsy. Any habit that may cause the disease must be stopped and the condition observed, or treated by cryosurgery, surgery, or laser treatment.

Lichen planus

Lichen planus is a fairly common skin disease of unknown aetiology that may affect the mouth, causing white patches or ulcers. The dentist may carry out a biopsy and prescribe treatment with corticosteroid pellets, paste, or other medication.

COLD SORES

Blisters on the lips are usually caused by cold sores (recurrent herpes labialis) (*Fig. 10.5*). After a child has had primary herpes (see page 101), the herpes simplex virus lies dormant in the trigeminal nerve. In about one out of three patients the virus is occasionally reactivated, appearing on the lips as cold sores (fever blisters). Reactivation is caused especially by sunlight, other infections (for example, a cold) and menstruation. Blisters fill with pus before they scab and heal; antiviral creams containing acyclovir may be useful if used at the beginning of blister formation.

Blisters contain the infectious virus which can be spread to persons who are non-immune (that is to say, they have not had the primary disease themselves). DSAs should, therefore, wear gloves when working in the mouth (see also page 11).

BLISTERS IN THE MOUTH

Blisters in the mouth are sometimes a sign of serious skin disease. They may rapidly break down, leaving persistent mouth ulcers. Patients should be examined by a specialist.

Mucocele

This is a single blister usually inside the lower lip or in the floor of the mouth, which is produced by saliva escaping from a damage salivary duct and collecting beneath the mucosa. Mucoceles are treated by excision or cryosurgery.

SALIVARY GLAND DISEASES

Saliva is important for protection of the mouth against infection (including dental caries), lubrication of food before swallowing, and taste. There is a constant, small amount of secretion of saliva mainly from the submandibular gland. With the sight, smell, taste or thought of food, salivation is stimulated with a large outpouring of saliva, particularly from the parotid gland. Over 1ml/min of saliva is produced by stimulation from each gland.

CAUSES OF ENLARGED SALIVARY GLANDS
Parotid (mumps, Sjögren's syndrome, tumour, bacterial infection)
Submandibular (obstruction of duct by calculus, mumps, tumour, bacterial infection)

Fig. 10.6 *Diseases of the salivary glands, causing swelling.*

Salivary gland swelling

Diseases of salivary glands are usually the following (see *Fig. 10.6*).

Mumps

Mumps is a viral infection usually affecting children, with painful swelling of the parotids, trismus and fever. There is no specific treatment available. DSAs not having a history of mumps may be susceptible to infection (but not always).

Stone

Blockage of the submandibular duct by a stone causes painful intermittent swelling of a gland, particularly at meal times. The stone is surgically removed.

Tumours

These are usually benign and affect the parotids. They are surgically removed, but as they are closely related to the facial nerve removal can be difficult and dangerous, as it may cause facial paralysis.

Sjörgren's syndrome

This is an immunological disease affecting several glands as well as the salivary glands. The eyes and mouth become dry and infected. The patient usually suffers from rheumatoid arthritis (see 'dry mouth' below).

CAUSES OF DRY MOUTH
Psychogenic
Drugs (anti-depressants)
Salivary gland damage (radiotherapy, Sjögren's disease)
Dehydration (diabetes)

Fig. 10.7 Factors that may lead to dry mouth.

DRY MOUTH

Causes of dry mouth are shown in *Fig. 10.7.*

Dry mouth may predispose to increased caries, thrush, bacterial infection of the salivary glands (sialadenitis), difficulty with eating and swallowing, and loss of taste. Patients with dry mouths should, therefore, be instructed in preventive dental care and oral hygiene, and given antifungal drugs and artificial saliva.

Conversely, sialorrhoea (excessive saliva) is a rare phenomenon, often in the imagination of the patient.

11. Pain

Pain is a sensation that can vary in severity, for example, from the mild transient discomfort caused by knocking an elbow against a hard surface, to the severe persistent pain caused by pulpitis. Also, pain in some areas, such as mouth and genitals, can often be much worse than pain elsewhere, as for instance from a boil on the back. The reaction to pain varies significantly between individuals and is altered by age, psychological and emotional responses, fatigue and other factors. Thus, some patients do not complain about pain following tooth extraction, whereas others complain bitterly even about a little discomfort. While they may be physical reasons for these differences, the patient's psychological make-up plays an important role.

CAUSES OF PAIN IN THE MOUTH AND FACE

Pain in the mouth is usually caused by caries, pulpitis or dental abscess, although other inflammatory problems, injury or tumour, may also be responsible (*Fig. 11.1*). Diseases of the jaws, temporomandibular joints, sinuses, salivary glands, throat, blood vessels or nervous system may also cause pain around the mouth. Some patients have pain because of psychological reasons.

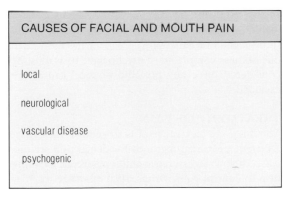

CAUSES OF FACIAL AND MOUTH PAIN
local
neurological
vascular disease
psychogenic

Fig. 11.1 Causes of facial and mouth pain.

CAUSES OF PAIN RELATED TO TEETH AND SINUSES

1. Early caries in dentine, a lost or leaking filling; exposed dentine at the tooth neck, or from fracture of the crown.
   Features: Intermittent, sharp pain produced by hot, cold or sweet substances, relieved on removal of stimulus.
   Other features: Caries or lost filling; dental hypersensitivity.
   Treatment: Restoration.

2. Pulpitis (pulp inflammation), usually due to caries.
   Features: Intermittent, severe, throbbing pain that comes on spontaneously, worsened by hot or cold stimuli but not relieved on removal of the latter.
   Treatment: Analgesics and endodontics.

3. Dental abscess (periapical).
   Features: Persistent, severe, throbbing pain, worsened by touching or biting on the affected tooth. The affected tooth is non-vital because of caries or trauma.
   Other features: Swelling of gingiva or face; possible fever; lymph node enlargement.
   Treatment: Root treatment, incision and drainage, or extraction; analgesics.

4. Periodontal abscess (lateral).
   Features: As for dental abscess, but the tooth is usually vital; there is also chronic periodontitis.
   Other features: Swelling of gingiva.
   Treatment: Incision and drainage, curettage, or extraction; analgesics (page 108).

5. Pericoronitis (inflammation of the flap of tissue over a partially erupted tooth, *Fig. 9.14*).
   Features: Persistent, dull pain, worse on biting; obvious tenderness and swelling of the gum flap.
   Other features: Trismus, bad taste and breath; sometimes fever; lymph node enlargement.
   Treatment: Irrigation of the area with chlorhexidine; application of astringents; antimicrobial agents (metronidazole or penicillin); analgesics; extraction if problems persist or recur.

6. Dry socket (infected with loss of blood clot following extraction).
   Features: Persistent dull pain with tenderness in the area, starting two to three days after extraction.
   Other features: Bad taste and breath.
   Treatment: Irrigation with warm saline or chlorhexidine; dressing gently with, for example, Whitehead's varnish, Alvogel, or Debrisan (page 147); analgesics.

7. Sinusitis.
   Features: Persistent, dull pain, worsened by mov-

ing the head or when lying down and sometimes on biting. It may follow a cold.

Other features: Nasal discharge, blocked nostrils.

Treatment: Decongestants, antibiotics; analgesics.

NEUROLOGICAL DISEASE

The trigeminal nerve is distributed through its three main branches — ophthalmic, maxillary and mandibular — to most parts of the mouth and face. Therefore, diseases affecting this nerve can cause pain in the mouth, face, or both. Some of these are:

Trigeminal neuralgia

This affects older people, with recurrent attacks of severe stabbing pain; patients usually need treatment with drugs (carbamazepine), or blocking of the nerve using cryosurgery (cryoanalgesia).

Disseminated sclerosis

This causes paralysis or patches of occasional anaesthesia in different parts of the body, as well as pain.

Herpes zoster (shingles)

This is caused by reactivation of the chicken-pox virus, which usually remains in the nerves supplying sensation to the skin throughout life after the attack. Shingles causes severe pain, a rash, and mouth ulcers if the trigeminal nerve is affected.

VASCULAR DISEASE

Spasm and dilatation of arteries supplying blood to the face and head may cause headaches or facial pain. Migraine is a condition of this kind, affecting women in particular, which may be precipitated by stress or some foods. At first there are symptoms related to vision (for example flashes of light), followed by a severe headache lasting hours or days and made worse by bright light; there is also an accompanying feeling of sickness and vomiting. Drugs to prevent attacks are available.

PSYCHOGENIC DISORDERS

There are three main types of facial pain that may have a psychogenic basis, which respond well to sympathetic handling and antidepressant drugs. It is always important to make sure that there is not a physical cause underlying the patient's pain.

Temporomandibular pain dysfunction syndrome

This is a common problem (especially among young women), with discomfort in the temporomandibular joint (TMJ) or muscles of mastication, and 'clicking' from the joints with or without limited mouth opening. The patient may have certain neurotic habits (for example chewing the end of a pencil), or suffer from psychosomatic disease. Few patients have evidence of disease in the TMJ; some may have imperfect occlusions. Most of these cases resolve either spontaneously without treatment, or after treatment with antidepressants, occlusal rehabilitation, use of various splints, exercise or rest.

Burning mouth syndrome

This is a less common problem, affecting older women in particular. The complaint is of a persistent burning sensation usually in the tongue, but examination reveals no abnormality. A few patients prove to be vitamin-deficient, but often the symptom appears to arise because of cancer phobia.

Atypical facial pain

Middle-aged and elderly women are usually affected by this pain, which appears to be a sign of depression. There is a persistent dull pain, over the upper jaw especially, and the patients often make repeated visits to the dentist insisting that their teeth are the cause of the problem.

Other psychogenic symptoms

Many complaints appear to have a psychogenic basis, including some types of dry mouth, discharge and spots in the oral mucosa. If a patient has more than one of these complaints, a psychogenic basis must be considered once any possible physical causes are excluded.

TREATMENT OF PAIN

The best way to treat pain is to remove the cause. Different treatment methods for dental pain are discussed below. Reassurance and sympathetic handling help to control pain. Drugs, such as analgesics, may be needed, but in some cases more serious medical or surgical treatment may be required. In severe pain that is unresponsive to drugs it may be necessary to block the nerve with an anaesthetic or by freezing it with a cryoprobe.

ANALGESICS

Aspirin (acetylsalicylic acid) is still one of the best painkillers available for adults, but not for children. Having been in use for many years, its safety in most situations is established and the occasional side effects are well known. Since it inhibits blood platelet function and may slow down the mechanism of blood clotting, it should not be given to any patient with a bleeding tendency. Occasionally, it causes bleeding after extraction. It also irritates the stomach lining and should not, therefore, be given to patients with peptic ulcers. Some patients are particularly sensitive (allergic) to aspirin.

Paracetamol is safer for children. It is also a good alternative for any patient in whom aspirin is contraindicated. It is almost as effective as aspirin, but more expensive. Paracetamol can be dangerous if an overdose is taken, as it may damage the liver.

Non-steroidal anti-inflammatory agents (NSAIDs), such as ibuprofen, are popular but expensive and may cause gastric irritation. Codeine may be required if the pain is too severe to be controlled by aspirin, paracetamol or NSAIDs. This is a powerful analgesic, but its main disadvantage is that it can cause constipation.

Morphine, omnopon and pethidine are dangerous drugs of addition, hence they should be used only as premedication for in-patients, to control severe post-operative pain or pain associated with cancer.

12. Anaesthesia and Sedation

Most dental procedures are carried out on highly sensitive tissues. Effective pain control is necessary to enable a patient to tolerate such operations. Patients may be given local anaesthesia to make an area numb and insensitive to pain without affecting the other senses (analgesia), or general anaesthesia to produce loss of all sensations, including consciousness.

DENTAL LOCAL ANAESTHESIA

Painful sensations from dental structures are directed to the brain along specific nerve pathways (see Chapter 2), where they are interpreted as pain. Deposition of local anaesthetic solutions around any of these nerves, or their branches, temporarily stops them from conveying painful messages to the brain. After some time, the effect of the local anaesthetics wears off, and nerve impulses return to normal. In the early days of local anaesthesia, naturally occurring cocaine was the only drug available but, apart from being dangerous, its effects were rather unpredictable. Synthetic agents used nowadays produce reliable and safe effects. Two are in common use: lignocaine and prilocaine. Other anaesthetic agents, such as mepivicaine and bupivicanine, are available and work in exactly the same way, but they are not as popular probably due to their higher cost. Lignocaine, most widely used, is supplied as a 2% solution, and prilocaine as a 3% or 4% solution.

Dental injections are administered into an area which is richly supplied with blood vessels. This means that the injected drugs are rapidly absorbed into the blood stream and eliminated from the body through the liver. Because of the rapidity with which anaesthetic agents are removed from the injected area, plain lignocaine anaesthesia does not last long enough for most dental procedures. To overcome this problem, adrenaline is added to the injected solution. This produces vasoconstriction of the area, reduces the blood flow, and prolongs the anaesthetic effects (concentration of 1:80,000). Plain 4% prilocaine is also fairly rapidly taken up into the circulation. Felypressin may be added instead of adrenaline to prolong anaesthesia. Felypressin has the advantage over adrenaline in that it has no effect on the heart or blood pressure. Patients with heart disease or high blood pressure may be advised to avoid adrenaline; therefore 3% prilocaine with felypressin is a useful alternative.

Dental equipment in local anaesthesia

Dental anaesthetic solutions are supplied in sterilised glass cartridges which have a rubber diaphragm at one end and a rubber plug at the other. Each cartridge contains either 1.8ml or 2.0ml of injectable solution (*Fig. 12.1*). The cartridge is loaded into a dental syringe with a screw-on, double-ended needle attached to it. The end of the needle projecting into the syringe pierces the rubber diaphragm of the cartridge. Pressing the syringe plunger pushes down the rubber plug at the other end of the cartridge, expelling the solution from the needle (*see Fig. 12.1*).

If an injection is accidentally made into the lumen of a blood vessel, drug reactions are far more likely to occur. Nowadays, many dentists avoid such problems by using self-aspirating cartridges for their dental syringes, designed such that, by discontinuing an injection, the rubber plug at the end of the cartridge recoils from the injection pressure, draining a small amount of fluid back into the cartridge. If the fluid contains blood, this indicates that the needle is

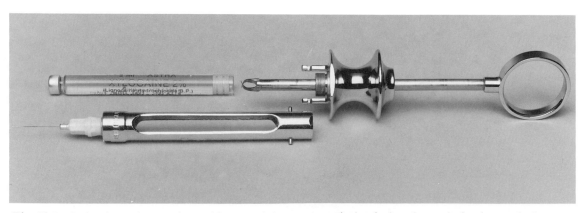

Fig. 12.1 *Aspirating syringe and cartridge containing an anaesthetic solution, for use in local anaesthetic injections.*

positioned inside a blood vessel. Thus, before the injection is continued, the needle position is readjusted and another aspiration test performed. A similar effect may be produced by using an Aspirating Syringe (*Fig. 12.1*).

Needles used nowadays are disposable, for single use only. Dental anaesthetic cartridges and needles should, therefore, never be used twice, as transmission of serious diseases (such as hepatitis or AIDS) may occur. Sharp syringe needles and glass cartridges should be disposed of in rigid containers designed for that purpose. (They should never be placed in ordinary waste, as they present danger to refuse collection personnel.)

Administration of local anaesthetics

Local anaesthetics can be administered in two different ways: by topical application to mucous membrane or skin, or by injection. Injections provide the necessary level and extent of anaesthesia required for most dental procedures. Topical applications result in the anaesthesia of only a very small area of soft tissue surface. Teeth cannot be anaesthetised by topical application.

Topical application

The anaesthetic agents used for this purpose are lignocaine, amethocaine, or benzocaine, and are available as sprays, pastes, gels, solutions or lozenges/pastilles. The lozenge/pastille is primarily used to give temporary relief from painful conditions of the oral mucosa. The other preparations may be used to provide a small degree of anaesthesia on an area of mucous membrane. This may be required for small incisions into its superficial layers, for releasing pus from an abscess, or for producing a small area of anaesthetic tissue through which a syringe needle may be passed painlessly.

Local injections

Several types of injections may be used. Each has its benefits and disadvantages. The dentist selects the type to be used according to the nature of treatment undertaken, the length of operating time required, the degree of anaesthesia necessary for the operation, and anatomical factors, such as the porosity of the bone which encloses some of the dental nerves (*see Fig. 12.3*). The types of injections are as follows (*Fig. 12.2*):

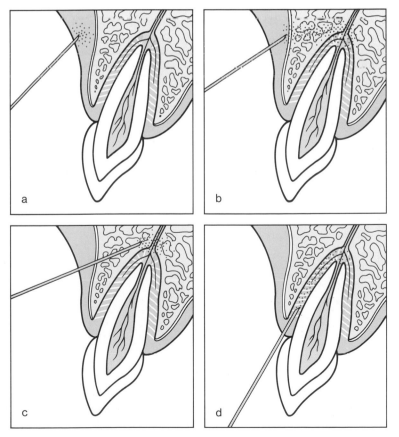

Fig. 12.2 *Types of local anaesthetic infections: (a) infiltration, (b) dental infiltration, (c) intraosseous, (d) intraligamentary.*

- Infiltration, to produce soft tissue anaesthesia only.
- Dental infiltration, to produce anaesthesia of individual teeth.
- Regional block, to produce anaesthesia of an entire area supplied by a major nerve trunk (see Fig. 12.4).
- Intraosseous, where the anaesthetic is deposited directly into the bone surrounding a tooth.
- Intraligamentary, where the anaesthetic is forced into the periodontal ligament of a tooth to produce anaesthesia.

Infiltration injections

For an area of soft tissue or skin, the anaesthetic solution is simply injected into the required area. This may be necessary in order to suture a skin or intraoral wound, or to remove a soft tissue lesion. The anaesthetic acts directly on the fine, terminal branches of the nerves, thereby making the skin or tissue supplied by these nerves numb and insensitive to pain.

Dental infiltration injections

These are used to anaesthetise teeth for conservative or endodontic treatment. The syringe needle is passed through the oral mucous membrane from the buccal or labial side, and the solution is injected so that it lies in contact with the surface of the bone covering the relevant root apex. The soft tissue in this area will rapidly become insensitive, as in soft tissue infiltration. In addition, after a short time the anaesthetic solution penetrates the pores of the bone and ultimately reaches the dental nerves which enter the apical foramen of the tooth in the injected area. Thus, the pulp of that tooth as well as the buccal gingiva will become insensitive.

The effectiveness of dental infiltrations in producing pulpal anaesthesia is obviously dependent upon the thinness and porosity of bone. The bone surrounding mandibular molars and premolars is dense and not very porous, therefore dental infiltrations will not anaesthetise the pulp of these teeth. Mandibular canines and incisors are susceptible to dental infiltrations, as the bone on their labial sides is very thin and porous. In children, all maxillary and deciduous teeth of both jaws may be readily anaesthetised by dental infiltration.

Regional block injections

Anaesthetic solution is deposited around a main nerve trunk. This blocks all impulses from the area that the nerve supplies. The best example is the inferior dental nerve block: solution is deposited around the inferior dental nerve just after it emerges from the mandibular foramen on the inner surfaces of the ascending ramus of the mandible (*Fig. 3.21a*). Impulses from the lower lip and all mandibular teeth on that side are blocked from reaching the brain, all these structures being anaesthetised by a single injection. As dense bone around mandibular molars and premolars prevents anaesthesia by infiltration, an inferior dental nerve block has to be employed to anaesthetise these teeth. Aspirating syringes or self-aspirating cartridges should be used (page 126).

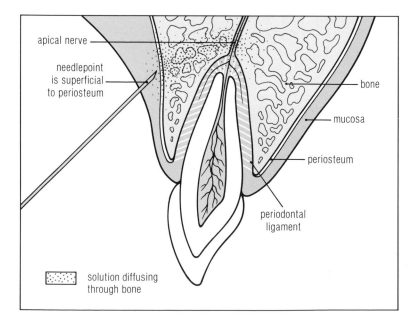

apical nerve

needlepoint is superficial to periosteum

bone

mucosa

periosteum

periodontal ligament

solution diffusing through bone

Fig. 12.3 An infiltration injection, in this example anaesthetising the tissues supplied by the apical nerve.

Intraosseous and intraligamentary injections

Special syringes are used to administer these injections. They are not used often, but are sometimes required when infiltration and regional block injections have failed to produce effective anaesthesia.

Local anaesthesia for conservation or surgery

As seen in Chapter 2, each tooth and socket with its surrounding gum receives a network (plexus) of nerves from three sources: one plexus supplies the tooth pulp (dental plexus), one supplies the buccal or labial structures (outer plexus), and one supplies the palatal or lingual structures (inner plexus) (*see Fig. 12.4*). For painless conservation of teeth, only the dental plexus needs to be anaesthetised. All maxillary teeth and mandibular incisors and canines may

be anaesthetised by a buccal or labial infiltration. Mandibular molars and premolars require an inferior dental nerve (regional) block.

For minor oral surgical procedures, including tooth removal, all three nerve networks must be anaesthetised. In the maxilla, this is achieved by a buccal/labial infiltration supplemented by a palatal infiltration. In mandibular incisor and canine repairs, all three nerve plexuses involved may be anaesthetised by a single injection. Anaesthetic solution injected around the main trunk of the inferior dental nerve will also surround the nearby lingual nerve. This will produce lingual plexus anaesthesia (lingual nerve), dental plexus anaesthesia (inferior dental nerve) and labial plexus anaesthesia (nerve branch of the inferior dental nerve); *see Fig. 12.4*. For

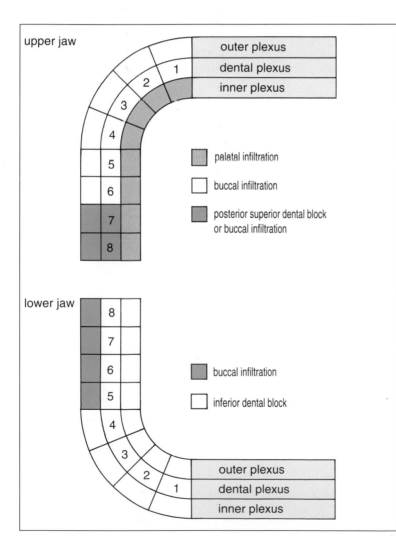

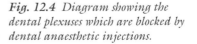

Fig. 12.4 Diagram showing the dental plexuses which are blocked by dental anaesthetic injections.

mandibular molar and premolar surgery, where the buccal plexus is not served by the mental nerve, an additional buccal infiltration injection is required (see page 52 for a more detailed discussion of these anatomical relationships).

Preparation

The sterile dental syringe is laid onto a sterile towel covering a tray or other suitable surface. Sufficient cartridges are disinfected by swabbing externally with a 70% alcohol solution containing 0.5% chlorhexidine. Once swabbed, the cartridges are placed onto the sterile towel. Cartridges stored in a refrigerator must be removed and allowed to reach room temperature before use. No further warming is needed.

There are long and short needles. Long needles are used for inferior dental nerve block injections, and short needles for infiltrations. The appropriate presterilised needle should have its outer case disinfected by swabbing with antiseptic, as described above, and placed with the other sterilised equipment.

Needle fracture is very rare nowadays, but may occur during dental injections. For this reason, a pair of 'Spencer Wells' artery forceps should always be ready for use, so that in case of fracture the dentist can immediately grip and withdraw the fractured end of the needle projecting from the tissue.

Some surgeons use a topical anaesthetic spray or paste for surface anaesthesia of the mucous membrane before needle penetration. Although this is generally unnecessary, it has a calming effect on many patients, especially children. Disinfection of the mucosa at the injection site with a cotton wool swab soaked in a 70% alcohol solution containing 0.5% chlorhexidine prior to needle puncture is advised.

Once the local anaesthetic injection is administered, the DSA offers the patient a mouthwash. Whilst the anaesthetic takes effect, the DSA must remain with the patient in case there is a reaction such as fainting, restlessness, or other emergency. Patients having just received an injection must *never* be left unattended. In the even of a reaction to the anaesthetic, the patient should be laid flat and the dentist summoned immediately. An exception to this rule is women at advanced stages of pregnancy, who should be turned onto their *side* not their back, because the weight of the fetus may compress the inferior vena cava, preventing normal venous return from the lower half of the body to the heart, leading to collapse and unconsciousness (see also Chapter 15).

After local anaesthesia

Patients may have meals, but should be warned of numbness of the mouth and lips for three hours, especially after an inferior dental nerve block.

They should avoid biting anaesthetised areas — tongue or lips.

They should avoid smoking until the anaesthetic has worn off.

GENERAL ANAESTHESIA

General anaesthetics produce a state of unconsciousness with total loss of all sensations. They are used where local anaesthetic injections are inappropriate or insufficient. General anaesthetics may be administered in general practice surgeries which are suitably equipped for emergencies. More usually, general anaesthesia is administered in hospitals or clinics by professional anaesthetists.

Patients undergoing short operations under general anaesthesia, for example, tooth removal or abscess drainage, may be treated as out-patients. Often, general anaesthesia is required where more complex procedures are planned, for which patients are admitted to hospital. They may be dismissed on the same day (day-case surgery), or after two to three days (short-stay surgery).

Indications

Acute infection or abscess

Local anaesthesia is both useless and dangerous if there is acute infection or an abscess at the injection site. Not only will the anaesthesia be poor, but there is great risk of spreading the infection extensively In some cases, it is possible to avoid passing a needle through or into an infected area by using regional block injection techniques. In other cases, this is quite impossible. Where drainage can be obtained, the patient may be offered pain relief and the infection controlled with antibiotics, so that after a few days local anaesthesia is possible. Occasionally, it is necessary to remove a tooth or drain an abscess immediately, as is the case when a dangerous level of infection is present. Under those circumstances, general anaesthesia has to be used; this, for many general dental practices, means referring the patient to hospital.

Long operations

To have many teeth removed at one sitting, using multiple local anaesthetic injections, would be intolerable for any patient. If it is not possible to remove the teeth under local anaesthesia, in small stages within a few days, then general anaesthesia is indicated. In addition, loss of all remaining teeth in one operation (dental clearance) could produce extensive bleeding which needs to be monitored, and this is best achieved by referring the patient to a suitably equipped hospital department. Major oral surgery obviously requires admission to hospital.

Difficult tooth removal

The length of time required to remove a tooth may make general anaesthesia necessary. The maximum surgical operating time under local anaesthesia is around thirty minutes. By the end of this period, the patient's tolerance is completely exhausted and thus it is unkind to plan longer operations. Also, after thirty minutes the effect of local anaesthesia subsides, and further injections are undesirable. These factors may make general anaesthesia necessary.

Treatment for the very young, anxious, or mentally handicapped patients

Very young children may require a general anaesthetic in order to have routine dental treatment or tooth removal, as their poor cooperation and understanding make local anaesthetic injections impossible. Extremely nervous adults or the mentally handicapped may render general anaesthesia necessary.

Contraindications

Medically unfit patients

General anaesthesia, especially in the dental chair, may be dangerous for patients who are not perfectly fit and healthy. Cardiovascular and respiratory diseases (including a common cold), and other diseases such as diabetes, render general anaesthesia in the dental surgery inadvisable. Under such circumstances, it is often better to perform the operation under local anaesthesia, or the patient should be referred to hospital for specialist management.

Drug treatment

Patients under therapy for psychological illnesses, and those under treatment for hypertension or on corticosteroids, should be referred to hospital for general anaesthesia. Patients on corticosteroids carry a special warning card which should be shown to the dentist.

Very large or obese patients

Obese patients do not tolerate general anaesthesia well, especially in the dental chair. This is particular-

ly the case if they also have a tendency towards alcoholism. Specialist treatment is therefore necessary.

Pregnancy

Dental out-patient general anaesthesia is not advised for pregnant women, especially those in their first or final trimesters of pregnancy. This is because damage to the fetus may result from any short period of oxygen shortage which could (but should not) occur during the procedure. The responsibility for both fetus and mother should be left to very experienced anaesthetists.

PREPARATION FOR OUT-PATIENT GENERAL ANAESTHESIA

Before the appointment for general anaesthesia is made, the dentist checks the patient's medical history to exclude drug treatment or diseases which would make the procedure undesirable or dangerous. Any previous anaesthetic experience of the patient should also be noted. Many establishments have a standard medical history questionnaire which the patient (or parent) completes. The DSA should check that the history has been taken for any patient prior to admission, and that the questionnaire is up-to-date and has been fully answered. Any relevant medical history, including pregnancy or allergies, must be brought to the dentist's attention before any dental procedure takes place. The patient or parent must sign a consent form, giving permission to the dentist and anaesthetist to carry out anaesthesia and operation. Every patient should attend accompanied by a responsible adult and warned in advance not to drive, cycle or operate any machinery for the remainder of the day. Patients should not consume food or drink for at least four hours before general anaesthesia.

The above factors must be double-checked and any discrepancies reported to the dentist immediately. At the time of anaesthesia, dentures, outer clothing and jewellery should be removed. All necessary sterile equipment and instruments, radiographs and the patient's notes are laid out in the surgery. The nature of treatment or operation should be verified with the patient or parent before anaesthesia is administered.

During the operation, the DSA assists the surgeon in the usual way. Afterwards, the unconscious patient should be laid flat, turned onto one side and observed closely, especially with regard to keeping the patient's airway clear in order to ensure a normal recovery. When consciousness returns sufficiently, the DSA assists with mouthwash rinsing and gently removes any blood marks from the patient's face. Once recovered, the patient is assisted from the surgery to the recovery room, and is discharged only when able to walk unassisted, after bleeding has stopped and proper after-care instruction has been given.

Types of general anaesthetics

Types of general anaesthetic agents may be classified into inhaled and intravenous. For inhalation anaesthesia, gases or vapours are administered to the patient through a tube attached to the anaesthetic machine which regulates the gas mixture delivered. The inhaled gases are absorbed into the blood stream across the epithelium of the lung tissues. Intravenous anaesthetics are injected directly into the patient's blood stream. Both types operate by affecting the normal function of the brain. As the anaesthetic agents are eliminated from the brain tissue, recovery occurs.

In inhalation anaesthesia, it is important to ensure that the patient is not deprived of oxygen, as this may lead to death. Atmospheric air contains 20% oxygen; during inhalation, the oxygen level of the gases delivered to the patient should never fall below this level.

Inhaled agents
Nitrous oxide
This is slightly sweet-smelling gas which is non-explosive and non-irritant to the delicate nasal and lung passages, supplied in blue cylinders. As an anaesthetic it has little harmful effect on the respiratory system and no direct action on the heart. It is, therefore, an extremely safe agent, easily administered and rapidly eliminated from the body through the lungs at the end of the procedure. However, it is very weak and will only produce a sufficient degree of anaesthesia if inhaled in 100% concentration, excluding oxygen. The unconsciousness produced by this method is not due to the nitrous oxide but to the lack of oxygen. This dangerous practice is no longer employed.

Nitrous oxide has excellent analgesic properties. It is used as the basis for virtually all general anaesthetics, supplemented by more powerful agents such as halothane. Oxygen is also added to give the required 20% concentration. For some nervous patients, inhalation of 50:50 nitrous oxide/oxygen mixture produces control of pain and anxiety without loss of consciousness. This is called 'relative analgesia' (page 134).

Halothane
Halothane (fluothane) is a colourless, pleasant, sweet-smelling liquid, which is non-irritant when inhaled. It has powerful anaesthetic properties but weak analgesic effects, and thus complements the properties of nitrous oxide well, thereby forming a highly effective anaesthetic mixture. Halothane also produces muscle relaxation which enables the patient's jaw to be opened easily. Halothane liquid is stored in a vaporiser incorporated into the anaesthetic machine. The vaporiser has a regulator controlling the amount of vapour entering the gas mixture delivered to the patient. Halothane is delivered at a concentration of between 0.5 and 4%.

One problem is that repeated administration of halothane over a short period of time produces harmful effects in the liver, leading to jaundice. For this reason, the patient's previous anaesthetic exposure must be known, and repeated administrations over short periods of time must be avoided. Enflurane and isoflurane are similar to halothane, and are becoming increasingly popular as alternatives to halothane.

Oxygen
In order to deliver anaesthetic gases to a patient which contain at least the same amount of oxygen as inspired air, cylinders of oxygen are incorporated onto the anaesthetic machines. Oxygen cylinders are black with a white top.

Intravenous agents
Intravenous injection of drugs may be employed to produce two different results: general anaesthesia or sedation. For general anaesthesia, *methohexitone* is widely used. This belongs to a group of compounds called 'barbiturates' which have powerful sedative effects. Methohexitone acts rapidly, but sleep is of short duration. It has no analgesic properties, so the unconscious patient still reacts to painful stimuli, making a delicate surgical procedure impossible. For this reason, it is used in conjunction with nitrous oxide, oxygen and halothane, to produce rapid, pleasant induction of anaesthesia. Ketamine and propofol are popular alternatives to methohexitone for intravenous induction.

General anaesthetic apparatus
Two types of apparatus are in use for dental anaesthesia: continuous flow (Boyle, Quantiflex) and demand flow (McKesson, Walton) machines.

Continuous flow machines
These are designed so that gases from the nitrous oxide and oxygen cylinders flow continually though

the attached tube, delivering the gases to the patient. A mask is fitted to the end of the delivery tube and fits the patient's face. A nasal mask leaves the mouth accessible during anaesthesia. The concentration of nitrous oxide and oxygen is controlled by flow meters, one for each gas. The mixture then passes through the halothane vaporiser where the controlled amount of halothane is added. A rubber reservoir bag is incorporated to the delivery tubing of a continuous flow machine. The rate of flow of gases is continuous but breathing is an intermittent process. Whilst the patient is breathing out, via a spring-loaded expiratory valve close to the mask, the gases collect in the reservoir bag awaiting the patient's next intake of breath.

Demand flow machines

Demand flow machines, introduced in 1910 by the American dentist McKesson, were very popular in the early days of dental anaesthesia. They supply a regulated mixture of gases, including halothane, only as the patient inhales. Such machines have been largely superseded by the simpler and more accurate continuous flow machines.

STAGES OF GENERAL ANAESTHESIA

Administration of a general anaesthetic eventually produces unconsciousness. The type of anaesthetic agent determines how rapidly this is produced. The patient passes through several stages of anaesthesia before the required depth of unconsciousness required for surgery is reached. The stages are as follows:

1. **Analgesia:** Sensitivity to pain is decreased, but consciousness and cooperation are maintained.
2. **Delirium:** The patient is unconscious but shows spontaneous movement with excessive reaction to stimuli, including noise.
3. **Surgical anaesthesia:** The patient is unconscious and immobile. There are no eye movements, and when the eyelids are lifted the eyes are seen to be central.
4. **Respiratory arrest:** Too much anaesthetic paralyses breathing, and death soon ensues.

Modern agents act very promptly, making the above stages not so obvious. Intravenous anaesthesia is so rapid that the patient almost instantly reaches a plane of surgical anaesthesia. It must be remembered by all staff that *hearing* is the last sense to disappear before full unconsciousness is reached, although the patient may seem unconscious.

Hearing is also the first sense which returns. Therefore absolute quiet should be maintained during induction of anaesthesia and recovery.

PROCEDURES FOR GENERAL ANAESTHESIA

All necessary surgical equipment is sterilised and set out on a sterile towel covering a tray or other suitable surface, and allowed to cool. The instruments are covered by a second sterile towel which, during operation, is removed and used as a protective bib for the patient. Emergency drugs and equipment should be readily available and drug expiry dates checked. Suction equipment is checked to ensure that it is in good working order. The machine apparatus should also be tested to ensure that the gauges attached to the gas cylinders indicate the presence of sufficient oxygen and nitrous oxide. Spare cylinders must always be available. The halothane vaporiser is filled if necessary. Where intravenous agents are employed, expiry dates are checked, and sufficient presterilised syringes and needles are made available for the anaesthetist.

Most general anaesthetics are administered with the patient laying almost flat. With modern muscle relaxing agents (usually halothane) there is no need to prop the patient's mouth open before anaesthesia. Props are used, however, to hold the patient's mouth open during the operation. These may be sterilisable rubber blocks of different sizes or a metal Fergusson's gag, which hold the patient's mouth open by being wedged between the upper and lower teeth.

If an intravenous anaesthetic is to be used, the DSA may be required to apply pressure around the upper arm either by gripping it or with a tourniquet, in order to dilate the veins. This enables the anaesthetist to see and select a suitable vein for injection. When ready to inject, the tourniquet or grip on the upper arm is released and the injection site is swabbed with antiseptic. Afterwards, the DSA applies a dressing to the injection site.

The dentist will not commence the operation until the anaesthetist is happy with the depth of anaesthesia, as well as with the patient's general condition. As the dentist's hands are scrubbed and gloved, the DSA switches on and adjusts the operating light and position of the dental chair. The dentist then places a gauze mouth pack at the back of the patient's mouth, to prevent teeth or other debris from entering the airway.

A DSA without surgically scrubbed hands and not wearing rubber gloves does not handle sterile swabs or instruments. These must be selected by the dentist from the tray positioned in a convenient place or handed to the dentist by a second DSA who is surgically scrubbed and gloved.

As teeth or other tissues are removed, they are placed into a kidney dish or other suitable receptacle where they may be checked to ensure that the operation has been completed correctly. At the end of the operation, the anaesthetist stops the anaesthetic, and the prop and mouth pack are removed after having turned the patient onto one side. The DSA is responsible for the after-care, as discussed on page 131.

Out-patient general anaesthesia always involves several duties for the DSA. Many establishments have trained nurses or helpers attending, so that recovering patients are looked after properly whilst the DSA assists the anaesthetist and dentist.

CONSCIOUS SEDATION

Most patients are able to accept dental treatment in which any discomfort is numbed by a local anaesthetic. However, some patients are unable to tolerate this approach unless they are helped by *sedation*.

Conscious sedation involves the carefully-controlled administration of a drug which depresses the central nervous system sufficiently to make dental care acceptable whilst allowing verbal contact to be maintained. Thus, the patient does not become unconscious (unlike under a general anaesthetic).

Sedation techniques and dental procedures may be performed by the same person, but it is obligatory that such a person is suitably experienced and also that a second appropriate person is present throughout the procedure. This second person may be a suitably trained DSA who is experienced in

- Chairside assisting
- Monitoring the patient's clinical condition
- Providing efficient and appropriate assistance should any emergency arise

Neither sedation nor general anaesthesia should be administered unless (a) the appropriate equipment is available to provide it correctly, (b) essential resuscitation equipment is to hand (page 157), and (c) the dentist and DSA are fully trained in their use.

All patients about to receive conscious sedation (or general anaesthesia) must give *informed consent* beforehand. It is essential that they

(a) fully understand what is to be done
(b) receive written and verbal instructions about

what they must do before and after treatment, and
(c) sign a consent form (giving permission for sedation, local anaesthesia, and dental treatment).

Methods of conscious sedation in current use are:
1. Oral sedation
2. Inhalation sedation ('Relative Analgesia', or 'RA')
3. Intravenous (IV) sedation

Oral sedation

The drugs used currently are either *diazepam* or *temazepam*. The methods of use to be described are for adults; oral sedation is unsuitable for children.

Diazepam may be taken as either a single 10mg dose one hour before treatment *or* in three divided doses (5mg the night before treatment, 5mg on waking, and 5mg one hour before treatment).

Temazepam may be taken as a 30mg to 40mg dose (3 or 4 capsules) one hour before treatment.

Either method is simple and relatively safe, and may produce some beneficial forgetfulness of the procedure. However, the depth and duration of sedation is unpredictable, and some patients may not remember to take the dose at the correct time. The recovery time after sedation by diazepam may exceed 6 hours; temazepam does not have this disadvantage.

Inhalation sedation (relative analgesia; RA)

This type of sedation is achieved by administering a carefully controlled mixture of *nitrous oxide* and *oxygen* from a special RA machine which is able to limit the maximum output of nitrous oxide to 50%. The gas mixture is delivered to the patient *via* a dental mask.

Nitrous oxide has weak anaesthetic properties but a beneficial analgesic effect. At a concentration of 20% to 35% in oxygen it produces a state of detachment and sedation, with some analgesia, enabling treatment to be carried out. However, a *local* anaesthetic may also be necessary (which might have been unacceptable to the patient prior to sedation). The sedated patient remains co-operative and responsive to verbal instructions and is able to cough if necessary. However, success with the technique is very much dependent upon psychological reinforcement, and is particularly useful for children who have been suitably conditioned and who are responsive.

Procedure for inhalation sedation

The RA machine should be checked to make sure that it is working correctly, has sufficient nitrous oxide and oxygen in its cylinders (with full, spare, cylinders to hand), and is unobtrusive.

The patient's medical history is checked. Nasal obstruction (e.g. a head cold), significant heart or lung disease, early pregnancy, certain drugs, and poor co-operation each contraindicates inhalation sedation. Written and verbal instructions to patients should emphasise

Before treatment
- Eat as normal
- Avoid alcohol
- Take any usual medicines (tell the dentist about them)

After treatment
- The effect of the sedative gas rapidly wears off
- The patient will be fit to travel home
- Do not drive or cycle immediately after treatment
- Do not undertake, for at least two hours, any responsible duties or work involving machinery
- Follow any other instructions (e.g. after tooth removal — page 144)

The patient is made comfortable in a supine position and provided with protective eyewear.

The dentist explains about the special face mask and that the first gas (oxygen) feels cold. Later (as nitrous oxide is also introduced) the patient may have a sensation of warmth and a pleasant tingling feeling in hands, feet, and limbs. These sensations do not cause alarm if the patient has been told beforehand what to expect.

Satisfactory sedation has been achieved when the patient is relaxed and has slowed responses (such as delayed answers to questions, and blinking less often). Whilst the patient continues to inhale the appropriate gas mixture through the mask, a local anaesthetic is given if needed, and the dental procedure is completed. During the procedure:
- The patient's pulse and respiration is monitored
- Leakage of gases from the edge of the mask should be prevented
- Patients should be discouraged from breathing through the mouth and talking
- All waste gases should be discharged outside the building

These precautions are to achieve optimum control of sedation and to minimise harmful pollution of the ambient air in the surgery by nitrous oxide.

After the procedure is completed, patients are *not* allowed to breath normal air immediately. Instead, the dentist switches off only the nitrous oxide, and — leaving the mask in place — allows the patient to inhale pure oxygen for at least two minutes. The mask is then removed and the patient is allowed to recover completely, whilst being gradually raised to a sitting position. When fully alert the patient may leave the surgery.

During the entire procedure the DSA needs to remain in constant attendance at the chairside.

Intravenous sedation (IV sedation)

The drug *midazolam* is the currently preferred agent for intravenous sedation. It is available in glass ampoules, each containing 10mg of midazolam in 2ml of sterile aqueous solution. When about 2mg to 7mg have been injected intravenously in stages (see below), midazolam produces relaxation for about one hour and a state of sedation with memory loss (amnesia) for the first 20-30 minutes.

The sedation is thus achieved solely by the drug, with no need for any psychological reinforcement. The amnesia effect reduces any unpleasant memories. The patient may take a light meal up to 2 hours before treatment.

Disadvantages of intravenous sedation are that:

- The drug cannot be retrieved as a means of overcoming any problems which it may cause.
- The drug has no pain-killing properties, so a local anaesthetic is also necessary prior to treatment.
- The patient's ability to cough is suppressed, so water and debris must be kept out of the throat.
- The patient must be accompanied to and from the surgery by a responsible adult (see below).

Intravenous sedation is unsuitable if the patient:

- Has no responsible adult escort.
- Is unable to avoid responsible duties for 24 hours
- Is a child
- Is pregnant or breastfeeding
- Is dependent on alcohol or other drugs
- Has any diseases of the liver, kidneys, heart, or lungs
- Has any mental, psychological, or neuromuscular impairment
- Has glaucoma
- Is taking other sedative drugs
- Is taking cimetidine (e.g. for stomach ulcers).

Written and verbal instructions to patients who are to receive IV sedation should emphasise:

Before treatment
- Bring a responsible adult with you who is able to wait to take you home.
- Have a light meal no later than 2 hours before the appointment.
- Take any routine medicines normally but ensure that the dentist knows about them.
- Do not consume any alcohol within 24 hours of the appointment.
- Ensure freedom from all responsible duties for 24 hours after sedation.

After treatment
- Travel home with your escort, preferably by car (not on the pillion of a motorcycle).
- Rest at home for 24 hours, avoiding driving, cycling, drinking alcohol, and operating machinery (including mechanical kitchen equipment).
- Observe any other requirements (e.g. after tooth removal)

Procedure for IV sedation

Before the patient enters the surgery, checks should be carried out on the emergency equipment (Chapter 15) and on the equipment for sedation and the dental procedure (including the giving of a local anaesthetic). It is important to check that the expiry dates of the midazolam and its antidote, flumazenil, have not been passed.

The patient should go to the toilet immediately before coming into the surgery. In the surgery, all personal details need to be checked, together with the nature of the procedure (and consent form signed). It is wise to involve the escort in checking that the procedures to be followed after treatment are understood and can be implemented.

The patient is placed supine in the dental chair with legs uncrossed. Any dentures are removed and placed in mouthwash. Any contact lenses are removed, and eye protection is provided. If the patient's pulse and oxygenation of the blood is to be continuously monitored, the method will need to be explained.

The dentist selects a suitable vein in the patient's arm or hand to receive the injection. The DSA may be required to have the syringe ready, to compress the patient's arm to facilitate venepuncture, and to release the pressure as the midazolam begins to enter the vein. The midazolam is *slowly* injected in small amounts (increments) at a time with an interval of about one to two minutes between each increment.

Sedation has reached a satisfactory level when the patient is obviously relaxed, with slurred speech and impaired neuromuscular co-ordination. (Sedated patients miss when asked to touch the tip of their nose with the index finger of their free hand!) For most adults, satisfactory sedation is achieved with a total amount of from 3mg to 7mg of midazolam. Elderly patients are more sensitive to this and similar drugs, so the total amount needed may not exceed 2mg, and the intervals between increments need to be longer. In all patients, overdosage is prevented by injecting the midazolam in stages as described. If 10mg has failed to produce sedation, the procedure should be abandoned.

If the patient is properly sedated, the dental procedure can commence (as mentioned earlier, *local* anaesthesia may be needed). Afterwards, the patient rests for at least one hour after the final incremental dose of midazolam was given. When able to walk unaided, the patient may leave the surgery to be escorted home.

13. Tooth Removal and Minor Oral Surgery

Tooth removal is one of the oldest and most commonly performed surgical operations, frequently referred to as extraction. The following reasons may make this operation necessary:

1. Failure of conservative or endodontic treatment.
2. Advanced periodontal disease.
3. Dental abscess.
4. Caries, where conservation is not possible or acceptable to the patient.
5. As part of a prosthetics treatment plan.
6. As part of an orthodontic treatment plan.
7. Impaction, commonly affecting wisdom teeth.

TOOTH REMOVAL

Two methods of tooth removal are available. The usual method is called 'forceps' removal. The blades of forceps are forced down into the periodontal ligament, between the tooth root and the bony socket wall. The root mass is gripped firmly between the forceps blades and, by gentle but firm movements, the socket walls are expanded to permit delivery of the tooth.

The other method of tooth removal is to dissect the tooth from its socket surgically. This applies to impacted teeth which cannot be removed simply with forceps, or to fragments of teeth which are retained or buried in the jaw. Once surgically exposed, the tooth or root is delivered using forceps or elevators. Minor surgery is sometimes used to obtain tissue for diagnostic purposes (biopsy), to treat cuts and lacerations of the mouth or face, and to control certain types of periodontal disease.

Forceps

These are made from high quality steel which provides the necessary strength to withstand the forces applied when removing teeth. Many different patterns exist. Forceps consist of three parts: the blades, the hinge and the handles (*Fig. 13.1*). The blades should be sharp to facilitate placement onto the tooth root; the hinge should move freely, but must not be worn or loose. The handles are serrated to give a firm handhold to prevent slipping during use. The blades of forceps are made in a variety of sizes called 'gauges', so that their size may be matched to the root mass to be gripped (*Fig. 13.2*). Large blades are termed 'heavy gauge', and narrow blades 'fine gauge'.

Different teeth require forceps with particular characteristics. Straight forceps have simple blades, which grip single roots, in line with straight handles. They are used to remove upper canines and incisors (*Fig. 13.1*). For upper premolars, straight forceps cannot be used easily as the lower jaw prevents the forceps blades being places on the tooth properly. The handles of upper premolar forceps are curved, so as to span the lower jaw and allow the simple blades to be correctly placed. These are called 'Read's' forceps (*Fig. 13.3*).

Lower incisors, canines and premolars are all removed with the same type of forceps which have a

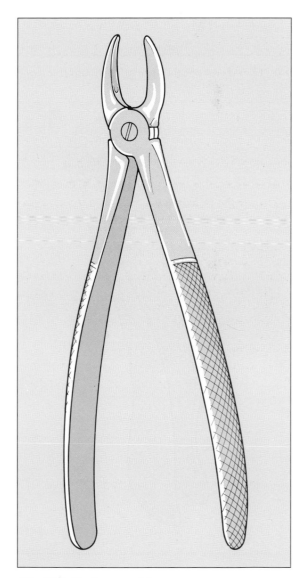

Fig. 13.1 *Tooth removal forceps.*

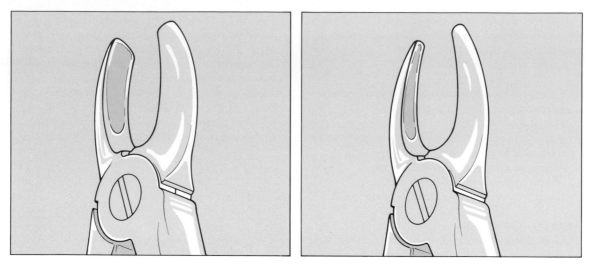

Fig. 13.2 Tooth removal forceps: heavy and fine gauge blades.

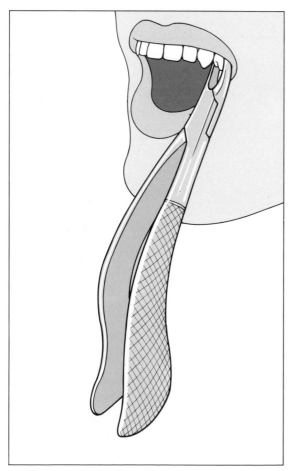

Fig. 13.3 'Read' forceps have two curves which permit the blades to be applied to the tooth correctly.

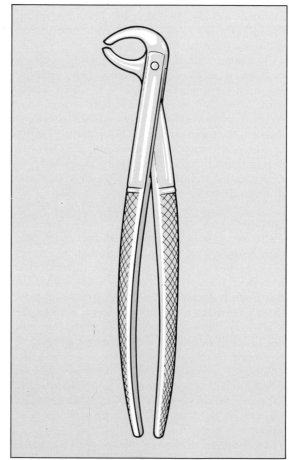

Fig. 13.4 Removal forceps for lower incisors, canines and premolars.

simple blade to grip the single root mass of these teeth. The blades are set at right angles to the handles (*Fig. 13.4*).

Lower molars viewed from the side have two root faces: one mesial and one distal. Thus, lower molar forceps have blades which are designed to grip both roots simultaneously, with the ends of the blades appearing pointed (*Fig. 13.5*). The point fits into the bifurcation between the roots. The handles of lower molar forceps are set at 90° to the blades.

Upper molars, viewed from the buccal side, also have two root faces, but on their palatal side there is only one root face. Thus, the blade design of these forceps must take this into account (*Fig. 13.6*). Furthermore, the handles are curved so that, as the blades are placed towards the back of the mouth, the handles span the lower jaw and teeth. This means that removal of upper right and upper left molars requires different set of forceps (*see Fig. 13.6*).

Elevators

Elevators are used to remove roots or impacted teeth from their sockets, where forceps are inappropriate. Many different types are available, usually identified by the surgeon's name who originally designed each particular pattern. Three of the more commonly used elevators are shown in *Fig.13.7*.

A Coupland's gauge is not, in fact, an elevator but a type of bone chisel. However, it enjoys popular use as a straight elevator for removing roots, or for driving into the periodontal ligament to dilate the bony socket and facilitate placement of forceps prior to tooth removal.

Warwick James' elevators have a slim shaft and a blade with a rounded end. The blade may be in line with the shaft or curved to one side. Hence they are made in sets of three: straight, left and right curved.

The direction of the curve is determined by a reference to the back surface of the blade (*see Fig. 13.7*).

Cryer's elevators have a sharp pointed triangular blade set so as to point to either the left or the right side of the shaft. The shaft of the elevator is also angled, so that it stays clear of the buccal tissues when in use. These elevators are very useful for removing lower molar roots, but they may be used elsewhere in accordance with the operator's preference.

Winter's elevators are similar to Cryer's, but with a T-shaped handle. They are no longer in common use because of the dangerous force they can generate.

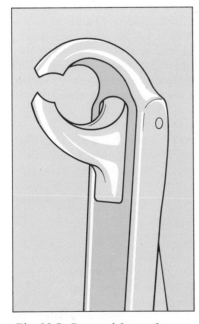

Fig. 13.5 *Removal forceps for lower molars.*

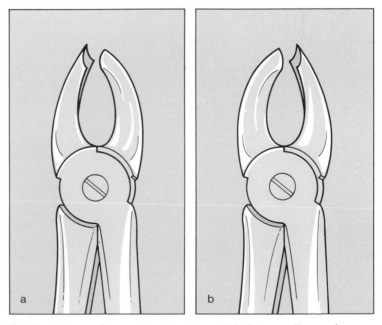

Fig. 13.6 *Removal forceps for (a) right and (b) left maxillary molars.*

jaws is complete. It is quite common for these teeth to have insufficient room to erupt completely. Frequently, an erupting lower wisdom tooth meets the distal surface of the second molar and becomes impacted against it. Often the distal cusps of this tilted tooth project through the gum into the mouth. Infection can spread beneath the gum into the bony space occupied by the impacted tooth. This causes pain and swelling (pericoronitis: see page 101). In order to prevent recurrences of pericoronitis, most impacted wisdom teeth are removed surgically.

Surgical removal of any painfully infected teeth or roots must be delayed until acute infection is controlled with antibiotics, otherwise a serious form of spreading bone infection (osteomyelitis) may result.

Retained roots

If, during the removal of a tooth with forceps, part of a root fractures and is left within the jaw, it may have to be removed surgically. Similarly, teeth which have had their crowns completely destroyed (for example, by caries), may have the retained roots removed surgically.

Removal of cysts

A cyst is an abnormal fluid-filled cavity with a definite lining of epithelial cells. Cysts slowly accumulate fluid and gradually enlarge. In the jaw, a cyst may develop at the apex of a tooth which has an infected, non-vital pulp (an apical or dental cyst), or in association with the crown of an unerupted tooth (dentigerous cyst). Other types of cyst are also found. If left untreated, cysts grow so large as to cause swelling and displacement of other adjacent teeth. They are, therefore, surgically removed.

Biopsy

A biopsy is the surgical removal of a piece of tissue for microscopic examination, in order to determine the nature of a disease. This is a very important procedure; it may be necessary to determine whether, for example, an ulcer in the mouth is cancerous or not.

Preprosthetic surgery

Before denture construction, it may be necessary to smooth and trim protruding or sharp areas of bone which forms the denture-bearing ridges, so that well-fitting, stable and comfortable dentures can be made. This operation is called 'ridge preparation' or 'alveoplasty'. If a plate of alveolar bone has to be removed the operation is known as 'alveolectomy'.

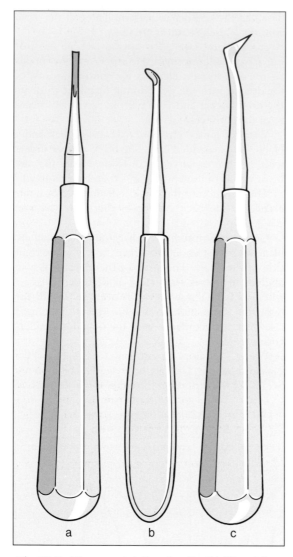

Fig. 13.7 *Elevators: (a) Coupland's; (b) Warwick James'; (c) Cryer's.*

MINOR ORAL SURGERY

All aspects of dentistry may require skilful minor oral surgery according to the planned treatment for a patient. Such operations include the following.

Removal of impacted wisdom teeth

Wisdom teeth (third permanent molars) are the last to erupt into the oral cavity, and usually do so between 17 and 21 years of age, when growth of the

Surgery in orthodontics

The orthodontist may require the assistance of the oral surgeon to expose an unerupted tooth. Once exposed, it may be left to erupt naturally or aided and directed into by orthodontic means.

Frenectomy is another operation which orthodontists may request. A very prominent labial frenum may be present between the upper central incisors, associated with an unsightly gap between these teeth (diastema). A prominent frenum may also require removal to enable effective toothbrushing or construction of an upper denture (see page 116).

Surgical endodontics are discussed in Chapter 6 and implants are described on page 151.

SURGICAL PLAN

Many of the above surgical procedure may be carried out under local anaesthesia in the dental chair. However, depending on the length of the operation, the medical state of the patient and the stress likely to be experienced under local anaesthesia, some of these operations are carried out in hospital operating theatres under general anaesthesia. All oral surgical procedure are carried out in accordance with a common plan or sequence, given below.

Raising a flap

First, an incision is made into the gum overlying the operation site with a scalpel. Where the gum overlies bone, the released areas of gum is raised from the underlying tissue using a periosteal elevator, and held to one side by a tissue retractor (*Fig. 13.8*).

Bone removal

This may be achieved with chisels and a mallet, or burs cooled with a stream of sterile 'isotonic' saline.

Isotonic saline is carefully prepared solution of salt (0.9% in water), which is compatible with body cells. If the solution is weaker or stronger than this, damage to living cells will occur. The use of chisels and mallets (*Fig. 13.9*) to remove bone in the conscious patient under local anaesthesia is rather unkind and rarely employed by most surgeons. Burs are normally used instead.

Delivery

Delivery of the exposed root or tooth is achieved by the use of suitable elevators or forceps.

Debridement

Any sharp bone spicules are removed with bone forceps (Rongeurs), and the margins of the socket are smoothed with a bone file (*see Fig. 13.9*). Small bone chips and filings are cleared from the socket and operative area by irrigation with sterile saline delivered from a Hunt's water syringe (*Fig. 13.10*).

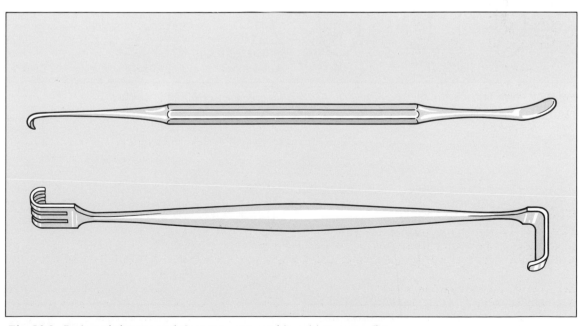

Fig. 13.8 Periosteal elevator and tissue retractor, used in raising a gum flap.

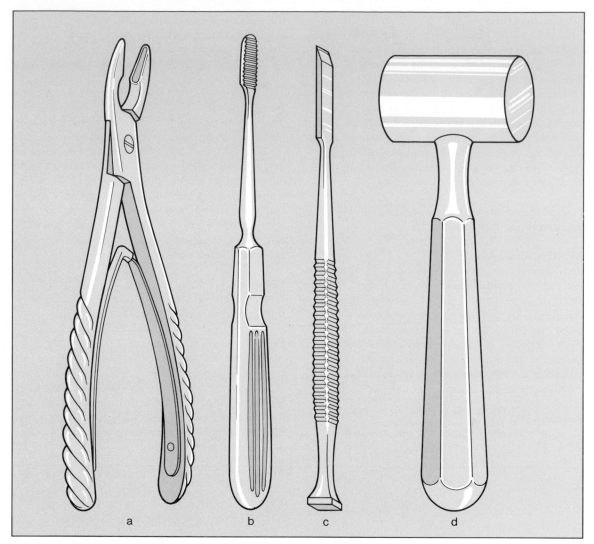

Fig. 13.9 *Bone instruments: (a) bone forceps (Rongeurs); (b) bone file; (c) chisel; (d) mallet.*

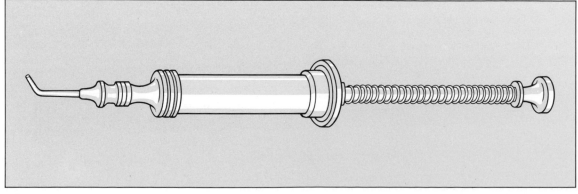

Fig. 13.10 *Hunt's water syringe used for irrigation.*

Suturing

Once the socket and operation wound are cleared of all debris, the flap is carefully replaced to its original position and held in place by inserting sutures (stitches) (*see Fig. 13.11*). Accurate positioning of the flap is facilitated by the use of dissecting forceps to hold the flap in place whilst the curved suture

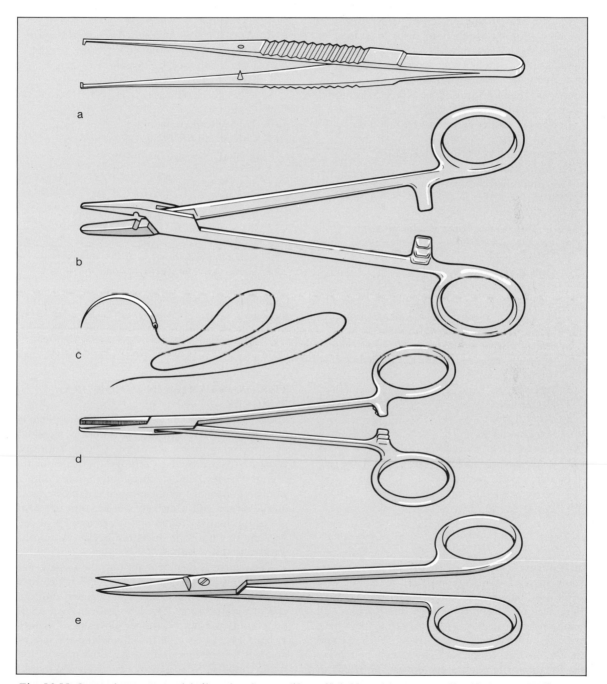

Fig. 13.11 *Suture instruments: (a) dissecting forceps; (b) needle holders; (c) suture needle; (d) Spencer Wells forceps; (e) scissors.*

needle, held in needle-holders, is passed through the tissues on either side of the wound. The suture is then knotted, and the ends cut with fine scissors. The materials commonly used for suturing are braided black silk or catgut. Black silk sutures are readily visible and are removed from intraoral wounds after seven days. Catgut sutures resorb (dissolve) after a few days. Suturing materials are made in a variety of thickness which is described by an '0'; the higher the number of '0's', the finer the material; 3/0 gauge is most frequently used for intraoral sutures, and the finer 5/0 gauge for suturing facial skin. Skin sutures are removed after five days.

In general, sutures perform three functions:

1. They control haemorrhage (bleeding)
2. They promote good healing
3. They restore normal anatomy

Tooth removal, suturing and haemostasis
Lay-up (with patient's records)
1. Moons probe
2. Topical anaesthetic
3. Local anaesthetic cartridge syringe, needle and cartridge
4. Selection of forceps: upper/lower molars, upper straights, upper/lower roots
5. Selection of elevators: Cryer's left/right/straight, Ash root, Coupland's chisels 1, 2, 3
6. Suction tips
7. Needle holders
8. Tissue forceps
9. Straight scissors
10. Spencer Wells artery forceps
11. Sutures: black silk 3/0, plain catgut 3/0
12. Sterile gauze swabs
13. Haemostats: Surgicel, Haemofibrin
14. Post-extraction advice

Instruments for out-patient surgical procedures
Many surgical items are supplied for single use, sterile and disposable. Towels, swabs, syringe needles, scalpels, aspirator tubes and sutures, all belong to this category. Non-disposable items have to be resterilised immediately before each use and include forceps, chisels and elevators. The following list of sterile equipment covers the needs of most dental surgical procedures performed on out-patients:

Basic surgical tray
Lay-up (with patient's records)
1. Moons probe
2. Local anaesthetic cartridge syringe, needle and cartridge
3. Bard-Parker scalpel handle and blade
4. Suction tips
5. Mitchell's osteotrimmer and periosteal elevator
6. Elevators: Warwick James' left/right/straight, Cryer's, Ash root, Coupland chisels 1, 2, 3
7. Austin tissue retractor
8. Kilner cheek retractor
9. Excavator
10. Rongeurs and bone files
11. Curved and straight mosquito forceps
12. Spencer Wells artery forceps
13. Needle holders
14. Straight scissors
15. Tissue forceps
16. Straight handpiece and surgical burs
17. Black silk suture 3/0
18. Hunt's irrigation syringe
19. Saline in galley pot
20. Sterile gauze swabs

The tray is covered with a sterile towel until needed.

THE DSA'S DUTIES IN MINOR ORAL SURGERY

For all surgical procedures, a sterile operative field is required. All necessary instruments must be sterilised by autoclaving or hot air. Sterile Cheatle's forceps (*Fig. 13.12*) are used to remove the instruments from the steriliser and lay them out, in order, onto a sterile towel on a tray or another suitable surface. Sterile swabs and a dish of sterile saline are also placed on the towel. A second sterile towel is placed over the tray until the operation begins. A mouthwash is also provided.

The patient is then brought into the surgery and seated comfortably in the dental chair. Any dentures are removed and stored in a dish of water until the end of the operation. The DSA and surgeon scrub their hands and put on rubber gloves (see Chapter 1, page 11). The sterile towel covering the instruments is fastened around the patient's neck with a sterile towel clip. The patient's hands should remain beneath it during the operation. The anaesthetic is then administered.

During the operation, the DSA assists the surgeon by passing instruments, using a sucker or swabs to keep the operation field clearly visible, and by retracting the lips, cheek or tongue as requested. Throughout the operation, where the patient is conscious, the DSA plays an important role in comforting and reassuring the patient. At the end of the operation, the DSA places the tray of instruments out of the patient's vision, covering it with the towel removed from around the patient's neck.

Postoperative instructions (page 146) are given and follow-up appointments made. Once bleeding is under control, the patient may be discharged with the dentist's permission. All instruments are then scrubbed absolutely clean and sterilised (page 12).

After-care

Following tooth removal or minor oral surgery, a patient must be given advice on after-care, and not discharged until bleeding has ceased. The patient should be advised not to interfere with the operation site during the ensuing 24 hours, to use the other side of the mouth for chewing, and to avoid excessive mouthrinsing. This is to prevent disturbance of the blood clot in the wound, which must be present for normal healing to take place. These points are summarised on page 54, together with information on bleeding, anaesthetic after-effects and discomfort.

In order to keep the operation site clean, a hot salt mouthbath is made up by the patient mixing one teaspoonful of salt in a tumbler of fairly hot water. A mouthful is held over the operation site until the fluid is cool, and then it is spat out. The patient continues until all the solution is used. This procedure should be undertaken four times daily. The use of such mouthbaths helps to keep the operation site clean and increases the blood supply to the area, which promotes good healing.

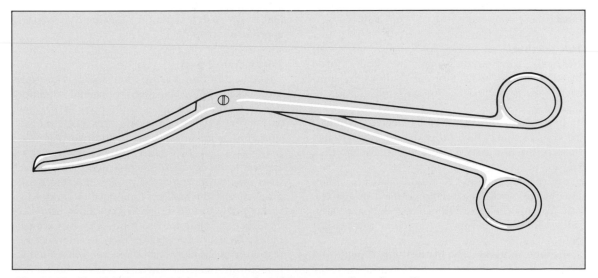

Fig. 13.12 Cheatle's forceps, used for removing dental instruments from the steriliser.

After tooth removal or minor oral surgery
To prevent the risk of blood clot loss, the following rules (1–6) must be observed:

1. No over-exertion or exercise.

2. No alcohol.

3. No rinsing for the rest of the day — after 24 hours hot salt water mouthwashes should be used.

4. Hot food, drinks and hard foods should be avoided.

5. Sitting in an overheated room should be avoided.

6. Tongue or fingers should not be placed in the socket.

Should bleeding occur, a clean, dry handkerchief is rolled up and bitten hard over the socket area for ten minutes.

In case of pain or complication, the surgery should be contacted.

POST-SURGICAL COMPLICATIONS
Postoperative recovery and healing progress normally in the vast majority of patients. Occasionally, however, some patients have to return to the surgery with severe pain or prolonged bleeding (haemorrhage).

Haemorrhage
Normally, when a cut is made into flesh, a little bleeding occurs which stops after about five minutes. This is normal haemostasis and consists of three stages:

In the first stage, the severed blood vessels undergo constriction which stops blood loss initially. Vasoconstriction lasts for several minutes and then relaxes.

In the second stage, blood platelets clump together to block the openings in the damaged vessels. When vasoconstriction of the first stage subsides, blood loss is now prevented by this platelet plug.

In the third stage, the platelet plug is reinforced by a firm, jelly-like clot (fibrin clot) formed at the site of injury, which prevents blood loss more permanently. Also, the clot forms the essential step towards repair of the wound during normal healing (see *Fig. 4.2*).

Clearly, tooth removal or any other surgical procedure must not be carried out on patients with bleeding diseases or those on anticoagulant therapy. Such patients must be referred to a specialist centre. The healthy patient who returns to the dental surgery with postoperative haemorrhage is very unlikely to be suffering from a rare bleeding disease. Most cases are likely to be caused by infection.

If the haemorrhage is within 24–36 hours after treatment pre-existing gingival infection may have interfered with the first stage of haemostasis; without vasoconstriction, the platelet plug and fibrin clot cannot form at the site of haemorrhage. A slow ooze of blood may continue for some hours, despite attempts to arrest the haemorrhage by biting onto a cloth pad.

The dentist usually puts a suture across the top of the bleeding socket, which compresses the tissue and artificially introduces vasoconstriction so that haemorrhage stops. The platelet plug and fibrin clot then form normally.

Bleeding can occur, however, two to three days after tooth removal or surgery, following apparently normal progress. The cause is usually secondary bacterial infection. Suturing plus antibiotic treatment will be required to control this type of haemorrhage.

Patients with bleeding from sockets or other surgical sites are naturally very anxious and must be seen without delay. The DSA can prepare for their arrival in the surgery by having their notes ready and laying up sterile suturing instruments *(Fig. 13.11)* and swabs as well as a local anaesthetic syringe and appropriate solution.

Postoperative pain
Excessive pain from a single tooth socket is known as 'dry socket'. This is an extremely painful condition, due to local inflammation of the bony socket wall, and develops two to three days after tooth removal. The cause is unknown, but it is through that infection plays a part. It is called 'dry' because the socket appears to be devoid of normal blood clot and the walls appear bare and dry. Factors which impede the production and retention of a normal blood clot in a socket predispose to a 'dry socket'. Such factors are disturbance of the formed blood clot by excessive mouth rinsing or bacterial invasion, or improper formation of blood clot which can occur following difficult tooth removal where excessive trauma has occurred. The condition more commonly affects

mandibular molar sockets, and these teeth are generally more difficult to remove than others. It was believed that the molar areas of the mandible had a poorer blood supply than the maxilla, and that this prediposed to inadequate blood clot formation, but it is now known that this is not so.

Pain control is achieved by analgesics (for example, soluble aspirin, paracetamol), and by local application of pain killing medicaments (obtundents) as a sedative dressing to the affected socket. Such dressings also protect the socket from collecting food debris which would delay healing.

A 'dry socket' is initially syringed with sterile saline, using a Hunt's syringe, to remove decaying blood clot and food debris. A dressing is then applied to the socket. An old remedy is a gauze dressing with a paste of zinc oxide and oil of cloves which was tucked into the socket. Many practitioners still favour this method of treatment. Such dressings need to be replaced every three days until the socket begins to heal satisfactorily, which may taken 2–3 weeks. Many proprietary pastes containing benzocaine, a topical anaesthetic, may be applied and repeated as necessary. Recently, a highly absorbent material resembling fine sugar grains (Debrisan®) has been used to treat 'dry socket' successfully. This material removes bacteria and other harmful substances from the socket, thereby promoting rapid healing as well as providing pain control. Two dressings 24 hours apart is usually all that is necessary. Hot saline mouthbaths are a useful adjunct to the management of 'dry socket'.

14. Prosthetics

Prosthetics is the branch of dentistry which deals with the replacement of missing teeth. In Britain, the term refers to the provision of removable appliances (dentures). In other countries, including the United States, crowns and fixed bridges are included. Patients who have had all their natural teeth removed (edentulous) will require complete dentures. When some teeth remain, partial dentures are needed (page 16).

COMPLETE DENTURES

These are usually constructed from a plastic material called 'polymethyl methacrylate' (usually known as 'acrylic'), which is coloured pink for the base of the denture. The acrylic artificial teeth are coloured in a range of shades to simulate natural teeth. The dentures are held in place by a film of saliva and the formation of a seal around the edges or peripheries of the denture, and are controlled by the muscles of the jaws, tongue and cheeks.

PARTIAL DENTURES

These are constructed from acrylic as well as from a metal alloy, usually cobalt and chromium, for additional strength. The dentures are held in place in the same way as complete dentures, but metal clasps are often added to anchor them firmly to the natural teeth.

FUNCTIONS OF DENTAL PROSTHESES

1. To restore the appearance of dentition.
2. To allow normal speech.
3. To facilitate mastication of food.
4. To maintain the correct relationship between upper and lower jaws.
5. To prevent drifting and overeruption of remaining teeth.

Where only anterior teeth are missing, appearance may be the most important reason for wearing a denture. As more teeth are lost, the other functions become important and hence should be explained to the patient.

Stages in the construction of dentures

The clinical procedures may only be carried out by a registered dental surgeon. Stages involving construction of dentures in the laboratory are carried out by the dental technician; these are shown in *Fig. 14.1*. It is the responsibility of the DSA to seat the patient comfortably in the dental chair, protect clothing with a bib, and have all materials and instruments available. The DSA also ensures that the patient's face is clean afterwards, and receives and despatches all laboratory work, with instructions, to the technician.

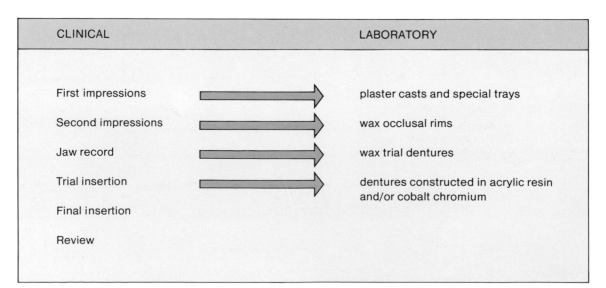

CLINICAL	LABORATORY
First impressions	plaster casts and special trays
Second impressions	wax occlusal rims
Jaw record	wax trial dentures
Trial insertion	dentures constructed in acrylic resin and/or cobalt chromium
Final insertion	
Review	

Fig. 14.1 Stages in the construction of dentures.

Examination and primary dental impressions

Before impressions are taken, examination of remaining teeth and oral mucosa in addition to the patient's medical/dental history (with particular reference to previous experience with dentures) is required. Radiographic examination may also be necessary. Primary impressions are subsequently taken. Upper and lower impression trays are selected from a range of standard shapes and sizes, known as 'stock' trays; these may be metal or plastic. Trays for taking impressions of jaws where natural teeth are present are box-shaped in cross section. Those for use in edentulous jaws are curved and more shallow.

The impressions are usually taken using alginate, plaster of Paris, or impression composition. Because alginate does not adhere to impression trays, and in order to prevent the material from lifting away from the tray when it is removed from the mouth, an adhesive is painted onto the tray surface. The solvent from this adhesive must be allowed to evaporate for three to four minutes before the alginate is placed in the tray. Some trays are designed with perforations or projecting fins to lock the alginate in position. It may be necessary to extend the trays with pink wax. The procedure of impression-taking in some patients occasionally stimulates the retch reflex and may cause the patient to vomit; a kidney dish should be at hand. For the procedure, impression trays and materials, pink wax, Bunsen burner, adhesive, a mixing bowl and spatula are required.

Following removal of the impression from the mouth, saliva, mucus, and other contaminants should be rinsed off the surface under running cold

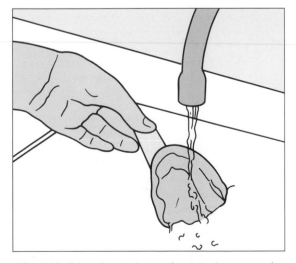

Fig. 14.2 Rinse impression under tap after removal from mouth.

water (*Fig. 14.2*). They should then be dipped or sprayed on all surfaces with a suitable disinfectant solution such as aqueous chlorhexidine 0.5%. Brief exposure to aqueous solutions do not have an adverse effect on the dimensional stability of alginate, but the impressions should not be left to soak for an extended period. Alginate impressions must then be wrapped in moist gauze and sealed in a polythene bag for rapid transport to the technician.

Cleaning impression trays

The technician will normally remove most of the alginate impression material from metal impression trays. Some dry alginate may remain, and to assist in its removal the tray is soaked in a solution of detergent for a few hours. Following this, the tray may be scrubbed and scraped to remove any remaining debris. Finally, the tray is put through the same sterilising cycle used for instruments. Trays which have been tried in the mouth, but not used, should also be sterilised. Disposable impression trays for single use are available, and are recommended for use as part of a policy for controlling cross-infection.

Secondary impressions

These are taken in trays specially constructed to fit the patient's mouth, with the objective of producing more accurate impressions. The clinical procedure is similar to that for the primary impressions. Green stick compound may be used instead of wax to modify the tray, and the impression may be taken using alginate, zinc oxide/eugenol paste, or an elastomeric material.

Recording the jaw relationship

In order that the biting surfaces of the dentures contact each other in a similar way to that of the natural teeth, the relationship (occlusion) of the upper and lower jaws must be recorded on wax occlusal rims, also known as 'record blocks'. The wax blocks are adjusted using a wax knife heated in a flame, to indicate to the technician the positions of the teeth. The vertical dimension of the lower part of the face, and hence the amount of jaw separation, can be measured using either a Willis gauge or a pair of dividers. Also, a wax knife, pink wax, shade and mould guides and an occlusal plane indicator are laid up.

The blocks are then sealed together, with the jaws in their natural position. The relationship between the upper jaw and the temporomandibular joint can be recorded at this stage, using a face bow. The DSA may be required to assist the dentist in positioning the face bow over the joint.

The colour and shape of the artificial teeth are selected and annotated on the laboratory prescription. This will also include details of the design of partial dentures. The casts and wax records are then returned to the technician, who sets the casts on an articulator (a hinged instrument designed to reproduce some of the jaw movements).

Lay-up
1. Bunsen burner
2. Wax knife
3. Willis gauge or dividers
4. Pink wax
5. Occlusal plan indicator
6. Shade and mould guides

The trial stage
Wax trial dentures are returned from the technician and positioned in the patient's mouth; the fit and occlusion are checked. An important part of this visit is to confirm with the patient that the appearance is satisfactory. When both dentist and patient are satisfied, the wax dentures are returned to the technician to be processed in acrylic resin. A further trial stage may be necessary if a metal partial denture is being provided.

Lay-up
1. Bunsen burner
2. Wax knife
3. Pink wax
4. Willis gauge or dividers

Fitting the dentures
The dentures are inserted in the patient's mouth. The occlusion and articulation are checked using articulating paper or wax, and any necessary adjustments are carried out using an acrylic trimming bur or a carborundum stone.

Finally, the patient will wish to examine the appearance of the dentures and may ask the DSA's opinion, which must be given with caution. It must be realised that new dentures may involve significant changes in the patient's appearance, and this may not always be acceptable initially. An encouraging and positive attitude can be most helpful.

Lay-up
1. Acrylic trimming burs and stones
2. Articulating paper
3. Polishing agents
4. Pressure-indicating paste
5. Face mirror

Review appointment
If there are difficulties with the dentures, rectification may involve adjustment of the dental occlusion or the pink acrylic bases (the review is a subsequent appointment). Instruments and materials are similar to those used for insertion of the dentures.

Advice to the patient
The DSA should be familiar with any recommendations which the dentist wishes the patient to follow. These may include:

Dentures

Practice is necessary to learn to wear new dentures.

The lower denture will always feel much looser than the upper.

Small mouthfuls are better at first, cutting the food into small pieces.

If speech alters, it will correct itself rapidly.

Wearing dentures for the first two to three nights helps the mouth to get used to them.

Dentures should be left out at night after the first two or three nights, always keeping them in cold water to prevent distortion.

Dentures need thorough cleaning at night using toothpaste, water and a denture brush (cleaning agents will not be necessary on new dentures).

They should be cleaned over a towel or basin of water, so that they don't break if dropped.

A lower denture being cleaned should not be held by the ends — it may break.

New dentures will probably cause sore spots during the first day or two. If this is so, leaving the dentures in for one or two hours before attending the surgery enables the sore spots to be seen by the dentist who can then ease the pressure.

Disabled patients may require special advice and provision of toothbrushes with large handles which may be gripped more easily.

OTHER DENTURES

Immediate dentures

These are inserted in the mouth immediately after removal of the teeth which they replace. Their advantage is that the patient is not left without teeth for any length of time, and the artificial teeth can be placed in the natural position. In addition, the denture protects the healing socket. One or more teeth may be replaced by the denture. The patient should be advised to:

- Wear the denture continuously for twenty-four hours
- Remove the denture after this period for rinsing
- Avoid vigorous mouthrinsing
- Return in case of undue postoperative pain or haemorrhage
- Arrange for a review appointment

Dental implants

Conventional bridges, and partial and complete dentures are supported by the natural teeth and the oral mucosa. However, implants in the form of a screw or cylinder may be placed in the jaw bone to support replacements for missing teeth (*Fig. 14.3*). The bonding of living bone to a synthetic implant is known as *osseointegration*. Dental implants are made of either titanium (a metal) or hydroxylapatite (a ceramic) and may be used in the following ways:

- A single implant to support a crown replacing one missing tooth
- Two or more implants to support a fixed bridge replacing several teeth
- Two or more implants to support a removable complete overdenture

Successful osseointegration depends upon:

- The choice of an implant which has been carefully and precisely manufactured
- A sterile operating field during the placement of implants
- An absence of pressure on the implant during a healing period of three to six months
- An appropriately designed superstructure
- Excellent oral hygiene

Obturators

These are dentures which have been modified to replace soft and hard tissues missing because of a congenital cleft palate, a post-surgical defect or trauma. Their function is to assist in normal speech and mastication, prevent food and drink from pass-

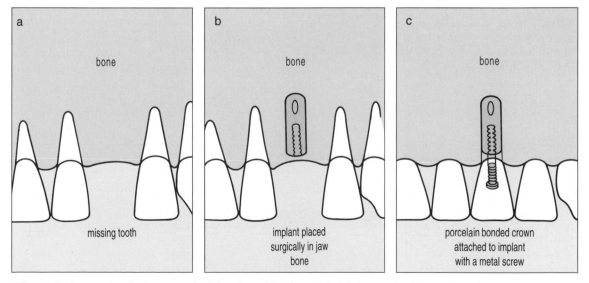

Fig. 14.3 *Stages of replacing a tooth with a dental implant. (a) Missing tooth. (b) Implant placed in jaw bone. (c) Porcelain bonded crown attached to implant with a metal screw.*

ing into the airways, and improve appearance. The clinical procedures are similar to those for complete dentures. The impression stage may require special techniques which may be uncomfortable for the patient if material enters deeply into the defect.

PREVENTION OF CROSS-INFECTION

Hepatitis B and AIDS are infectious diseases caused by viruses which are present in the blood and possibly also the saliva of infected patients. Patients who have symptoms of the diseases may be identified and must be treated in accordance with the recommended guidelines. However, dental patients who are carriers may be otherwise fit and healthy but still capable of transmitting the virus. It is, therefore, necessary to take precautions to protect the dentist and DSA from direct infection and also other patients from cross-infection via contaminated instruments.

In addition, the dental technician is potentially at risk through contaminated impressions, occlusal rims, wax trials and dentures which have been in the patient's mouth. It is, therefore, becoming common practice to regard all patients as being infection risks. All clinical items which have been in the patient's mouth and which are to go to the dental technician must therefore be thoroughly washed, disinfected with chlorhexidine, and wrapped before dispatch.

MATERIALS IN PROSTHETIC DENTISTRY

Impression materials may be:

Elastic: hydrocolloids, elastomers

Rigid: impression compounds, plaster of Paris, zinc oxide/eugenol paste.

Elastic materials
Hydrocolloids
Alginate

This is the most commonly used impression material in dentistry. In order to understand its handling characteristics, the nurse should know its basic chemistry. The main constituents of alginate impression materials are:

- Sodium or potassium alginate (active ingredient)
- Calcium sulphate (active ingredient)
- Trisodium phosphate (retarder)
- Diatomaceous earth (filler)
- Colouring and flavouring agents

When the powder is mixed with water, a non-reversible reaction takes place resulting in the formation of an insoluble, firm but elastic gel of calcium alginate. The reaction is summarised in *Fig. 14.4.*

As with other chemical reactions, this will take place rapidly if the temperature is high, and slowly if the temperature is low. The proportions of powder to water should be as recommended by the manufacturer. The mixing procedures are shown in *Figs. 14.5–14.8.*

Reversible hydrocolloids

These are jelly-like materials which soften in a warm water bath and set as they cool. Cooling takes place in the mouth, using impression trays with cold water flowing through them. The materials may be used in prosthetics or for crowns and bridges. The impression must be cast immediately.

Elastomers

These materials have the advantage that they are stronger than hydrocolloids. Also, they do not

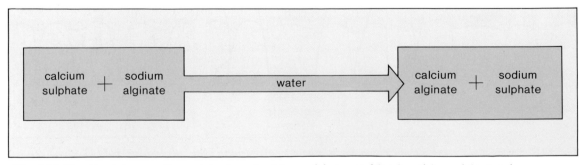

Fig. 14.4 Reaction between sodium alginate and calcium sulphate, resulting in calcium alginate gel.

undergo significant dimensional change if the impression is not cast immediately. Fast setting silicones may also be used for bite registration.

Rigid materials
Composition
This is a thermoplastic material; that is, it is softened and made plastic by an increase in temperature. It hardens as it cools down to body temperature. There are two types, both composed of a mixture of waxes, gums, resins and filler, known as impression compound and tracing sticks.

Impression compound is supplied as red or brown cakes and used for first impressions in trays. The material softens in a waterbath between 55 and 60°C.

Tracing sticks are green in colour and are used to modify trays or compound impressions. They soften over a flame.

Plaster of Paris
This is dehydrated calcium sulphate, a material which sets to a hard mass when mixed with water,

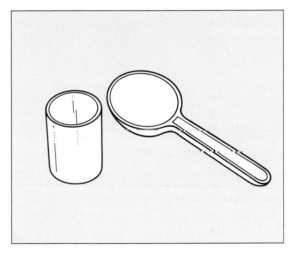

Fig. 14.5 Use the measures supplied by the manufacturer of the brand of alginate.

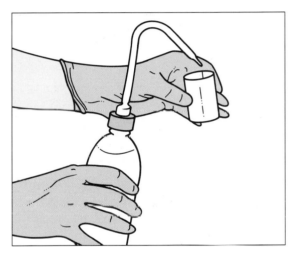

Fig. 14.6 Use room temperature water.

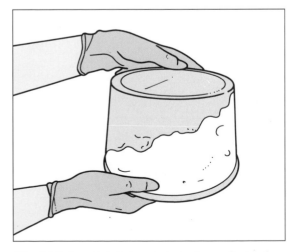

Fig. 14.7 Invert container twice to loosen the powder which may be packed down.

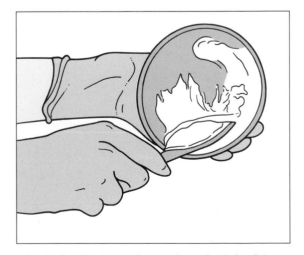

Fig. 14.8 Mix vigorously in a clean plastic bowl for recommended time — usually 30–60 seconds.

153

expanding as it sets. For dental use, an anti-expansion salt (potassium sulphate) and a retarding agent (borax) are added to the powder or water. The mixing procedure is as follows:

1. The manufacturer's recommended proportions are used.
2. Room temperature water is placed in a clean flexible bowl.
3. The powder is sprinkled on the water.
4. The mixture is allowed to absorb for 20 seconds.
5. The mixture is spatulated carefully for 30 to 40 seconds, avoiding air bubbles.

The material is rigid and not strong when removed from the mouth. If it fractures, the pieces should be carefully retained and wrapped with the impression.

Zinc oxide/eugenol paste

Equal quantities of the two pastes are mixed with a spatula on a slab until a uniform colour is achieved. The paste adheres to skin, and this can be prevented by applying petroleum jelly to the patient's lips. An orange-flavoured solvent is available to clean away the set material

Functional impression materials and tissue-conditioning materials

These are used beneath dentures to which they adhere, thereby recording an impression over several hours or days. They also provide a 'cushion', allowing damaged tissues to heal. They are presented in a powder and liquid form which, when mixed according to the manufacturer's proportions, form a plastic mass which flows initially, but becomes elastic inside the mouth.

15. Medical Emergencies

The most common medical emergency in the dental practice is fainting. However, the DSA must have a firm understanding of other less common medical complications that may arise, and should be aware of the correct management procedures for each disorder.

LOSS OF CONSCIOUSNESS
Fainting
This is the most common cause of loss of consciousness. It is normally of short duration, and frequently affects young adult male patients. Factors that predispose to a fainting attack are: (a) Anxiety concerning dental pain and/or the ensuing dental procedure. (b) Fatigue, if the patient has been unable to sleep due to severe pain. (c) Lack of food, as a result of problems with eating. (d) High temperature and humidity in the dental surgery.

Clinical features
A fainting attack develops rapidly; initially patients often feel dizzy, disorientated and nauseous. They become pale and the skin feels cold and clammy. Before loss of consciousness, the pulse is slow and weak.

Management
The patient's head should be lowered immediately by adjusting the chair to the supine (i.e. lying flat) position. Any tight clothing should be loosened, and smelling salts may be of value. All patients who have fainted will spontaneously recover consciousness within a minute or so. Once conscious, the patient should be reassured and, whenever possible, the dental procedure postponed. A patient who fails to recover consciousness within two minutes may have a serious medical problem (see page 55).

Myocardial infarction
This usually occurs in patients who have hypertension or a history of angina pectoris, previous myocardial infarction, or stroke.

Clinical features
Patients complain of a crushing chest pain which can radiate to the left arm and side of face. They become breathless, nauseous, and may lose consciousness.

Management
If the patient is still conscious, a 0.5mg tablet of glyceryl trinitrate should be placed beneath the tongue or the patient given two puffs of glyceryl trinitrate spray (eg Nitrolingual®). If the pain does not diminish, a 50:50 mixture of nitrous oxide and oxygen should be administered; this will relieve the pain and mildly sedate the patient. A tablet of aspirin should be given — this improves the patient's long term prognosis.

Cardiac arrest
This is when the heart either stops or suddenly contracts in an erratic manner (ventricular fibrillation). It is clinically characterised by loss of consciousness, absent pulse and respiratory movements. Cardiopulmonary resuscitation is required to maintain cardiac output and oxygenation of the blood and hence of the tissues.

Cardiopulmonary resuscitation
1. Lay the patient on a flat surface, preferably on the floor.
2. Ensure the airway is clear — remove dentures and oral debris. Pull the chin back and blow into the mouth or nose — if the airway is clear, the chest will rise.
3. If these is still no pulse begin external cardiac massage by compressing the sternum about two inches at a rate of 60 compressions per minute (80 per minute if only one attendant is available).
5. After every 5th or 6th compression, blow into the mouth or nose (2 blows every 15 compressions when only one attendant is available).
6. If there is no pulse after 15 minutes, it is likely that the patient is dead.

Hypoglycaemia
This is a problem of insulin-dependent diabetics. The patients have low levels of blood glucose, either because they have taken their daily dose of insulin without having had a meal, have delayed taking their next meal or have exercised vigorously.

Clinical features
Diabetics usually known when they are hypoglycaemic, and are likely to inform the dentist accordingly. These patients are often irritable or aggressive, have an easily detectable pulse, and have moist skin.

Management
If conscious, four lumps of sugar should be given orally. However, if the patient loses consciousness, the dentist may give intravenously, 20ml of a sterile 20% solution of glucose. An ambulance should be called.

Important Note: Although hyperglycaemia can also cause loss of consciousness, hypoglycaemia is the usual cause. Thus, administration of insulin should only be carried out when it is certain that hyperglycaemia is the cause of the loss of consciousness.

Anaphylaxis

This severe disorder occurs 30–60 minutes after the oral administration of a drug (usually penicillin) to which the patient is allergic. It can also arise within a few minutes if the drug is given intravenously or intramuscularly.

Clinical features

At the early stages, the face is flushed and the patient complains of a generalised itchiness or tingling (paraesthesia) and the skin can develop generalised wheals (urticaria). This is quickly followed by breathing difficulty and nausea. The skin become pale, cold and clammy, and the patient loses consciousness.

Management

Management must be prompt, otherwise irreversible brain damage will result. Unlike fainting, the patient will not recover within a minute or so, therefore anaphylaxis must be suspected when a drug has been given in the preceding thirty minutes.

The patient should be laid flat; the dentist should administer 1ml 1 in 1,000 adrenaline intramuscularly, and 200mg hydrocortisone hemisuccinate intravenously. The DSA should call an ambulance and, in the meantime, oxygen should be administered to the patient.

Corticosteriod insufficiency (hypotensive crisis)

This arises in patients suffering from Addison's disease, or after having taken corticosteriods over long periods of time (for example, for rheumatoid disorders). A hypotensive crisis is characterised by unconsciousness with a rapid fall in blood pressure, and may be precipitated by stress (for example, due to infection, trauma, general anaesthesia, or anxiety concerning the dental treatment).

Clinical features

Patients become pale and rapidly lose consciousness. There is a marked fall in blood pressure.

Management

The patient should be laid flat with the legs raised; 200mg hydrocortisone hemisuccinate must be given intravenously by the dentist, and an ambulance called. Oxygen may be administered to the patient until medical assistance arrives.

Stroke (cerebrovascular accident)

This can arise in elderly patients with a history of hypertension, previous myocardial infarction, angina, stroke or diabetes mellitus. Stress can be precipitating factor. Patients may rapidly lose consciousness although weakness of a limb or part of the face is a more likely presentation. Oxygen should be administered and an ambulance called.

SEVERE CHEST PAIN

This is most usually caused by angina pectoris, myocardial infarction or anxiety. Unlike myocardial infarction (see above) an attack of angina is usually short-lasting and does not lead to unconsciousness. Patients with a history of angina usually carry glyceryl trinitrate tablets or spray. It is often worthwhile to ask the patient to have a tablet or the spray available in case an angina attack develops during dental treatment. A tablet or two puffs of spray given sublingually usually quickly relieves the pain.

SEIZURES AND FITS
Epileptic attack (grand mal)

An epileptic attack can arise spontaneously, although it may be precipitated by withdrawal of anticonvulsant medication, alcohol, drugs (such as tricyclic antidepressants), fatigue, infection, stress, or menstruation.

Clinical features

A grand mal attack consists of several stages: initially, patients become irritable and develop a headache (aura phase); spasms and loss of consciousness follow (tonic phase). Uncontrolled jerking subsequently begins (clonic phase), which usually stops after a few minutes (recovery).

Management

Patients in the tonic phase should be placed on the floor (if possible), and protected from hurting themselves during the clonic phase. A patent airway should be maintained. Most patients recover within five minutes. If the spasmodic movements do not stop the dentist may administer intravenous diazepam (up to 20μg/kg at a rate of 2.5mg/30sec) and an ambulance must be called.

Asthmatic attack

As a result of anxiety, infection or administration of

drugs (such as aspirin or penicillin), asthmatic patients may become acutely breathless.

Management

Patients should be reassured and given their normal antiasthmatic drugs (usually a bronchodilating inhaler). They should *not* be laid flat, as this only accentuates the breathing difficulty. Oxygen is administered; if the attack persists, the dentist may give intramuscular adrenaline (1ml or 1 in 1000 solution). The DSA should call for medical assistance.

ACUTE RESPIRATORY OBSTRUCTION

Although this is a consequence of severe dental infection, haemorrhage or trauma, mechanical obstruction by a foreign object (endodontic instrument, fragment of tooth or filling material) is the most common cause of respiratory blockage in the dental practice. Coughing usually dislodges the object. However, if this is of no help, the Heimlich manoeuvre should be carried out (*Fig. 15.1*). If this still fails to dislodge the object, the patient should be referred to an Accident and Emergency unit so that the object be removed by endoscopy.

EMERGENCY KIT

In view of the medical emergencies that can arise in the dental practice, an emergency kit (*Fig. 15.2, overleaf*) should be an essential part of the dental equipment. It is of paramount importance that the DSA recognises each item in the kit, and ensures that all the drugs are undamaged and have not passed their expiry dates. DSAs may also consider attending a First Aid training course.

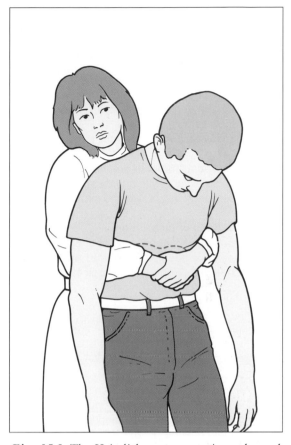

Fig. 15.1 *The Heimlich manoeuvre is a planned action designed to expel an obstructing bolus of food from the throat, by a sudden thrusting of the fist into the abdomen, between the navel and the rib cage, so as to force air up the trachea and thus dislodge the obstruction.*

POSSIBLE EMERGENCY KIT COMPONENTS

Airway maintenance
a) Suction apparatus — powered and portable (independently powered)
b) Simple airway adjunct (eg pocket resuscitator mask with valve)
   Oropharyngeal airways sizes 1, 2, 3
   Suction catheters sizes 6, 10 FG
c) Cricothyroid puncture needle (1)

Oxygen and artificial ventilation
a) Portable oxygen with appropriate valves, metering and delivery system
b) Self-inflating bag, valve and mask with oxygen enhancement facility

Maintenance of circulation
a) Disposable syringes — sizes 2, 5, 10ml (5 of each)
b) Disposable needles — sizes 21 and 23G (10 of each)
c) Disposable IV annulae — sizes 16 and 22G (5 of each)
d) Disposable IV infusion sets (2)
e) Scissors (1 pair)
f) Tourniquet, sphygmomanometer, stethoscope (1 of each)
g) Injection swabs

First line resuscitation drugs (minimum amounts)
a) Oxygen
b) Adrenaline 1mg in 1ml or 10ml (5 ampoules)
c) Lignocaine 1% (10ml) (5 ampoules)
d) Atropine 0.6mg (1ml) (5 ampoules)
e) Calcium chloride 14.3% (10ml) (2 ampoules)
f) Sodium bicarbonate 8.4% (50ml) (3 ampoules)
g) Glyceryl trinitrate tabs 300 micrograms (10)
   or Glyceryl trinitrate 400 micrograms per metered (1)
   sub-lingual spray

Second line drugs (minimum amounts)
a) Aminophylline 250mg (10ml) (2 ampoules)
b) Salbutamol inhaler 100 micrograms per metered dose (2 refills)
c) Chlorpheniramine maleate 10mg (1ml) (2 ampoules)
d) Dextrose 50% (50ml) (1)
e) Hydrocortisone 100mg (2ml) (5 ampoules)
f) Flumazenil 500 micrograms (5ml) (5 ampoules)
g) Naloxone 0.4mg (1ml) (5 ampoules)
h) Midazolam 10mg (5ml) (5 ampoules)
i) Suxamethonium 100mg (2ml) (5 ampoules)
j) Infusion solution
k) Dextrose 4%/saline 0.18% 500ml (2 packs)
l) Colloid solution 500ml (2 packs)
m) Diazepam solution (Stesolid®)

Fig. 15.2 Components of a possible emergency kit. (As recommended by the Poswillo Report, 1991.)

Index